OXFORD ONCOL

Vaccines for the Prevention of Cervical Cancer

O O L
OXFORD ONCOLOGY LIBRARY

Vaccines for the Prevention of Cervical Cancer

Revised Edition

Edited by

Peter L Stern

Professor of Immunology,
Paterson Institute for Cancer Research,
University of Manchester,
Manchester, UK

and

Henry C Kitchener

Professor of Gynaecological Oncology,
St. Mary's Hospital,
University of Manchester,
Manchester, UK

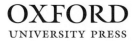

OXFORD
UNIVERSITY PRESS

OXFORD
UNIVERSITY PRESS

Great Clarendon Street, Oxford OX2 6DP

Oxford University Press is a department of the University of Oxford.
It furthers the University's objective of excellence in research, scholarship,
and education by publishing worldwide in

Oxford New York

Auckland Cape Town Dar es Salaam Hong Kong Karachi
Kuala Lumpur Madrid Melbourne Mexico City Nairobi
New Delhi Shanghai Taipei Toronto

With offices in

Argentina Austria Brazil Chile Czech Republic France Greece
Guatemala Hungary Italy Japan Poland Portugal Singapore
South Korea Switzerland Thailand Turkey Ukraine Vietnam

Oxford is a registered trade mark of Oxford University Press
in the UK and in certain other countries

Published in the United States
by Oxford University Press Inc., New York

British Library Cataloguing in Publication Data

Data available

Library of Congress Cataloging in Publication Data

Data available

Typeset by Newgen Imaging Systems (P) Ltd., Chennai, India
Printed in Great Britain
on acid-free paper by
Ashford Colour Press Ltd., Gosport, Hampshire.

ISBN 978-0-19-958863-3

10 9 8 7 6 5 4 3 2

Contents

Preface

Prophylactic HPV vaccines have the potential to revolutionize cervical cancer prevention by preventing the primary HPV infection that is the necessary cause. For the last 50 years, cervical screening, which relies on using cytology to detect pre-cancerous lesions which can be effectively treated, has been the mainstay of secondary prevention and has saved hundreds of thousands of lives. The technique of exfoliative cytology, developed by George Papanicolaou, has been possible because of the relatively easy access to the cervix, combined with a well-defined and lengthy pre-cancerous phase, providing ample opportunity to treat pre-invasive lesions. The advent of colposcopy enabled the conservative treatment of cervical intraepithelial neoplasia, which was both effective and fertility sparing.

These treatment principles were established before we understood the cause of cervical cancer. Epidemiology suggested an infectious aetiology; originally herpes simplex was suspected. By the late 1970s human papilloma virus became the prime candidate and with the identification of cancer-associated types in the early 1980s, it was Harold zur Hausen who suggested that HPV was the cause of cervical cancer. Over the next decade, molecular biology revealed the mechanism of HPV oncogenesis, and epidemiological studies using newly developed techniques of HPV testing, began to reveal the extraordinarily strong association between HPV infection of the cervix and subsequent cancer.

Immunologists began to unravel the immunological response to HPV infection, and the vision of developing a vaccine became a reality. The breakthrough came in the early 1990s with the discovery that the purified viral coat protein of HPV 16 could self-assemble into virus-like particles, which were capable of mimicking the virus.

These virus-like particles became the basis for the prophylactic vaccines which have been licensed and marketed over the last years, based on proven ability to prevent persistent infection, pre-cancer and, we assume over time, cancer.

This book marks the implementation of these vaccines. It is intended for a broad readership from researchers, healthcare professionals, and an informed public. It has been written by an authoritative group of contributors and is in four sections. The first section covers current prevention and treatment as a means of demonstrating where we are. The second deals with HPV and cervical disease, including both carcinogenesis and the epidemiological relationship, and concludes with how HPV testing can be utilized in clinical practice. The third section begins with an account of our current understanding of the immune response to HPV infection and how HPV infection is controlled. It then goes on to describe how the vaccines proved to be effective, confirmed by the results of pivotal global trials, which have led to the vaccines being approved, and finally the challenges of implementation in the real world. The final section looks ahead to the prospects for vaccines, which will protect against more multiple HPV types, for therapeutic vaccines, and in some ways the most important issue—how to get the vaccines to the women in the world who have the greatest need—those who live in the poorest countries with the highest disease rates.

Despite every attempt to keep the text lucid, there are inevitably, necessary scientific terms, which we have explained in a glossary that we hope will be useful.

Peter L Stern
Henry C Kitchener

Contributors

Adeola Atilade
University College Hospital,
London, UK

F Xavier Bosch
Servei d'Epidemiologia
i Resgistre del Càncer,
2ª Planta, Institut Català
d'Oncologia,
L'Hospitalet de Llobregat,
Barcelona, Spain

Loretta Brabin
Reader in Women's Health,
University of Manchester,
Manchester, UK

Xavier Castellsagué
Servei d'Epidemiologia
i Resgistre del Càncer,
2ª Planta, Institut Català
d'Oncologia,
L'Hospitalet de Llobregat,
Barcelona, Spain

Tanya Chawla
Senior Lecturer in Gynaecology,
University of Aberdeen
Medical School,
King's College, Aberdeen, UK

Margaret E Cruickshank
Consultant, Department of
Gynaecological Oncology,
Aberdeen Royal Infirmary,
Scotland, UK

Karin Denton
Consultant Cytopathologist,
Department of Pathology,
Southmead Hospital,
Westbury on Trym,
Bristol, UK

Henry C Kitchener
Professor of Gynaecological
Oncology,
St Mary's Hospital,
University of Manchester,
Manchester, UK

Julia E Palmer
Subspecialty Trainee in
Gynaecological Oncology,
Department of
Gynaecological Oncology,
Sheffield Hospitals
NHS Trust, Sheffield, UK

Sally Roberts
Senior Lecturer,
Division of Cancer Studies,
University of Birmingham,
Medical School,
Edgbaston,
Birmingham, UK

Richard BS Roden
Associate Professor,
Department of Pathology,
John Hopkins University
School of Medicine,
Baltimore, USA

CONTRIBUTORS

Silvia de Sanjosé
Servei d'Epidemiologia
i Resgistre del Càncer,
2ª Planta, Institut Català
d'Oncologia, L'Hospitalet de
Llobregat, Barcelona, Spain

**Rengaswamy
Sankaranarayanan**
Head, Screening Group,
International Agency for
Research on Cancer,
Lyon, France

Catherine Sauvaget
Screening Group, International
Agency for Research on Cancer,
Lyon, France

Margaret A Stanley
Department of Pathology,
University of Cambridge,
Cambridge, UK

Peter L Stern
Professor of Immunology,
Paterson Institute
for Cancer Research,
Christie Hospital NHS Trust,
University of Manchester,
Withington, Manchester, UK

John A Tidy
Consultant in Obstetrics
and Gynaecology,
Sheffield Teaching Hospitals,
Northern General Hospital,
Sheffield, UK

Sjoerd H van der Burg
Associate Professor,
Head of Laboratory
of Clinical Oncology,
Leiden University Medical
Center, Leiden,
the Netherlands

Patrick Walker
Consultant,
Department of Obstetrics
and Gynaecology,
Royal Free Hospital,
London, UK

Lawrence S Young
Professor of Cancer Biology,
Head of Division of
Cancer Studies, Cancer
Research UK Institute for
Cancer Studies,
University of Birmingham,
Medical School Edgbaston,
Birmingham, UK

x

Abbreviations

ADC	adenocarcinoma
AGE	advanced glycation end products
AIDS	acquired immune deficiency syndrome
AIN	anal intraepithelial neoplasia
APCs	antigen presenting cells
ASCUS	atypical squamous cells of undetermined significance
ASR	age-standardized rate
BCG	Bacillus Calmette-Guérin
BSCC	British Society of Cervical Cytology
CGIN	cervical glandular intraepithelial neoplasia
CIN	cervical intraepithelial neoplasia
CRPV	cottontail rabbit papilloma virus
CSP	Cervical Screening Programme
CT	Chlamydia trachomatis
CTLs	cytotoxic T cells
cVLPs	chimeric virus-like particles
DC	dendritic cells
DTP	diphtheria–tetanus–pertussis
EPI	Expanded Programme on Immunization
FDA	U.S. Food and Drug Administration
GNI	gross national income
GP	general practitioner
GW	genital warts
HBV	hepatitis B vaccine
HIb	Haemophilus influenzae b
HIV	human immunodeficiency virus
HLA	human leucocyte antigen
HPV	human papilloma virus
HPV HCII	HPV hybrid capture II
HR	high-risk

HR HPV	high-risk HPV
HR HPV PCR	HR HPV polymerase chain reaction
HSIL	high-grade squamous intra epithelial lesion
HSV-2	herpes simplex virus-2
IARC	International Agency for Research on Cancer
i.m.	intra-muscular
LBC	liquid-based cytology
LEEP	loop electrosurgical excision procedure
LLETZ	large loop excision transformation zone
LSIL	low-grade squamous intraepithelial lesion
MCM	mini chromosome maintenance
MCV	measles containing vaccine
MVA	modified vaccinia virus Ankara
NHS	National Health Service (UK)
NIP	national immunization program
NPV	negative predictive value
OR	odds ratio
PCTs	Primary Care Trusts
PPV	positive predictive value
QATs	quality assurance teams
Rb	retinoblastoma
RR	relative risk
RRP	recurrent respiratory papillomatosis
SCC	squamous cell carcinomas
SLP	Synthetic long peptides
STI	sexually transmitted infection
TA	tumour antigens
TCR	T cell receptor
Td/IPV	tetanus, diphtheria, polio
Th	T-helper
TIC	tumour-infiltrating cells
TT	tetanus–toxoid
TZ	transformation zone
VAIN	vaginal intraepithelial neoplasia

Glossary

Disease related	
Adenocarcinoma (**ADC**)	A glandular cancer arising from CGIN – accounts for 10–15% of cervix cancers
Adenosquamous carcinoma (**AdSC**)	Mixed carcinoma accounting for 2–3% of cervix cancers
Anal intraepithelial neoplasia (**AIN**)	Precancerous lesion arising from the anal epithelium
Atypical Squamous Cells of Uncertain Significance (**ASCUS**)	Bethesda classification of very low grade
Cervical (Pap) Smear	Cell preparation obtained by scraping cervix, placed on glass slide and graded for degree of abnormality by qualified cytoscreener
Cervical Glandular Intraepithelial Neoplasia (**CGIN**)	Precancer arising from glandular cells in the cervix
Cervical intraepithelial neoplasia (**CIN**)	Histological definition of pre-invasive cellular abnormalities in cervical epithelium
CIN 1 CIN 2/3	Low grade High grade
Colposcopy	Use of magnified image to identify location and grade of abnormalities of the cervix
Cytology	Use of exfoliated cells to identify any abnormality
Ectocervical lesions	Lesion visible entirely on outside of cervix
Endocervical lesions	Lesion is within cervical canal
Exfoliated cells	Surface cervical cells derived from scraping the cervix with a spatula or brush.
Genital warts (**GW**)	Benign warts caused by HPV 6/11 in the anogenital area
High grade squamous intraepithelial lesion (**HSIL**)	Bethesda classification of high grade cytological abnormality
Histopathology	Use of tissue sections to identify pathological changes
Hysterectomy	Removal of entire uterus (womb)
Large loop excision of transformation zone (**LLETZ**)	Popular methodology of excising CIN

Liquid based cytology (**LBC**)	Use of liquid preservative to achieve optimal presentation of cells on a slide
Low grade squamous intraepithelial lesion (**LSIL**)	Bethesda classification of low grade cytological abnormality
Mild, moderate, severe Dyskaryosis	Increasing degree of pre-invasive cellular abnormalities in cervical cytology
Negative predictive value	Proportion of cases that correctly predict a negative outcome
Positive predictive value	Proportion of cases that correctly predict an abnormality
Quality Assurance (**QA**)	Used to ensure agreed standards and consistent practice
Recurrent Respiratory Papillomatosis (**RRP**)	HPV6/11 driven, benign, but potentially dangerous because of airway obstruction
Squamous carcinoma of Cervix (**SCC**)	85% of cervix cancers that arise from CIN 3
Transformation zone (**TZ**)	Part of cervix at risk of developing squamous neoplasia
Triage	Process to separate individuals with different risks of disease
Vaginal intraepithelial neoplasia (**VAIN**)	Precancer of vaginal epithelium
Vulva intraepithelial neoplasia (**VIN**)	Precancer of squamous cells of the vulva

Virology related

BPV	Bovine papilloma virus
Capsids	The outer coat of the virus which encloses the viral genome (genetic material)
Capsomeres	Subunit of the capsids
Cell apoptosis	Programmed cell death often as a result of damage including events that may eventually promote cancer
Cell Senescence	Death through aging
Cellular immortalization	Unlimited prolongation of cellular lifespan
COPV	Canine oral papilloma virus
CRPV	Cottontail rabbit papilloma virus
Cytology/HPV testing-Sensitivity	Ability of a test to correctly identify a negative result
Cytology/HPV testing-Specificity	Ability of a test to correctly identify a positive result

Differentiating cervix epithelium	Process that produces the stratified layers of the skin overlying the cervix which is necessary for the life cycle of HPV
Epidemiology	Study of disease patterns as means to determine aetiology (cause of disease)
Genetic instability	Happens in cells where DNA repair mechanisms are inhibited
Genetic mutation	Changes in DNA sequences which can lead to altered function including the promotion of cancer
High risk HPV	Subset of HPVs identified with cervical cancer
Human papilloma viruses (**HPVs**)	Group of viruses that infect various epithelia of the body
Hybrid capture	Type of HPV test
Incident Infection	Newly acquired infection
Low risk HPV	Subset of HPVs not identified with cervical cancer
Malignant transformation	Changes in cell growth promoting cancer
Onco-gene, -protein	Product that is associated with cancer
Persistent infection	An infection that is not cleared by the immune system
Productive infection	Production of new infectious virus
ROPV	Rabbit oral papilloma virus
Telomeres	Ends of chromosomes which shorten with age
Transcription factor	Protein that controls the production of a specific RNA from DNA
Tumour suppressors	Products that act to control cell growth, inhibition can promote cancer
Viral episome	Viral genome copies in the cell
Viral integration	Viral genome is mixed with the host genome and replicates with the latter
Virus like particles (**VLP**)	Capsid like structures usually composed of L1 proteins and with no viral DNA
Virus particles	The infectious unit of the virus
Virus prevalence	The proportion of population who have a virus prevalence at a time point

Immunology related

Adaptive immunity	Production of specific antibodies/ T cells to fight disease and provide immunological memory to provide protection against any subsequent infection
Antigen presenting cells (**APC**)	Cells that efficiently present antigens to T cells for optimal and appropriate activation to generate useful adaptive immunity
B cells	Cells that produce antibodies
Cellular immunity	Innate and adaptive cellular effectors
Cytokines	Large group of molecules which have a plethora of functions including communication between immune cells and/or direct effects on virus infected cells (e.g. interferon)
Cytotoxic T cells (**CTL**)	Killer T cells able to destroy virus infected cells
Dendritic cells (**DC**)	Professional APC
HLA molecules	Tissue type of individuals important in antigen presentation
HLA-peptide complexes	The molecular complexes that are recognized by the T cell receptor
Humoral immunity	Production of antibodies
Immune Co-stimulation	Necessary set of signals for optimal activation of immunity
Immuno-dominant	Some parts of antigens are recognized preferentially e.g type specific epitopes on individual HPVs
Immunosuppression	Failure to mount a useful immune response
Innate immunity	Body's immediate defense against infectious agents
Interferon (**IFN**)	Molecules that inhibit viruses and virus infected cells
Neutralizing antibodies	Antibodies that can inactivate viruses
Peptide epitopes	Part of protein processed by APC and presented with HLA molecules to T cells expressing the specific TCR
Regulatory T cells	Subset of T cells which can limit adaptive immunity (eg control of autoimmunity or anti-tumour immunity)
T cell Anergy	Stimulation of specific T cells such that they are non responsive

T cell receptor (**TCR**)	Receptor of T cells e.g. recognizing viral peptides associated with HLA molecules
T cells	White cells that fight infections
T helper (**Th**) cells	Subset of T cells that organize other immune cells
Toll like receptors	Sensors expressed by innate and adaptive immune cells which respond to various molecules deriving from tissue damage or pathogens
Tumour antigen (**TA**)	Potential target for adaptive immunity (eg E6 and E7)
Tumour infiltrating lymphocytes	White cells found in a lesion or tumour which may be a mixture of CTL, T regulatory and other types

Vaccine and Clinical related

Adjuvant	Agent that boosts the immune response
Antigenicity	Property of a molecule that can be recognized immunologically
Booster immunizations	The requirement for further vaccination at a time after the initial immunization
Case control study	Compares abnormal cases with normal outcomes to identify associated risk factors
Confidence intervals	The margin for error around any result
Cross protection	Vaccine against one HPV type shows activity against another type
DNA vaccines	Vaccine based on DNA coding sequence for a protein
FDA	Food and Drug Administration
HIV/AIDS	Human immunodeficiency virus/ Acquired immune deficiency syndrome
IARC	International Agency for Research in Cancer
Immunization protocol	Specified regimen for vaccination in specific group of individuals
Immunogenicity	Ability to induce an immune response
Multivalent HPV vaccines	Vaccines that contain multiple HPV type VLPs
Power of study	Statistical prediction of ability to provide a degree of certainty regarding outcomes
Prophylactic vaccine	Vaccine to prevent infection and consequent disease

Risk estimates	Comparison of outcomes for a given risk factor in different populations (e.g. smoking and lung cancer; HPV infection and cervical cancer
Statistical analysis	Means to calculate degree of certainty of any result obtained
Therapeutic vaccines	Vaccine designed to treat established infection or its consequent disease
Type specific vaccines	Vaccines that protect against specific HPV type
Vaccine vectors	Bacteria or viruses genetically engineered to express e.g. L1 proteins
WHO	World Health Organization

Part 1

Prevention and current treatment

Chapter 1

The UK cervical screening programme

Karin Denton

> **Key points**
>
> - The Cervical Screening Programme (CSP) in the United Kingdom is fully integrated across the lifetime of a woman and across all clinical disciplines.
> - Cervical screening is estimated to prevent up to 80% of all cases of cervical cancer in the United Kingdom.
> - All aspects of the programme are defined by published specifications and standards.
> - The programme has high population coverage and is rigorously quality assured.
> - Liquid-Based Cytology (LBC) implementation will be complete in 2008.
> - Maintaining the protection currently offered by cervical screening while new technologies are implemented will be a challenge, but can be achieved.

1.1 History

The National Health Service Cervical Screening Programme (NHS CSP) in the United Kingdom evolved gradually rather than being implemented in its entirety. In fact, cervical cytology has been performed in the United Kingdom since the 1940s, but it was only in 1988 with the advent of computerized call and recall that population coverage rose and a true programme emerged. There are, in fact, four CSPs in the United Kingdom—in England, Scotland, Wales, and Northern Ireland and although there are subtle differences, all four are very similar. The NHS CSP covers England, and this chapter relates mainly to the English programme.

The incidence of cervical carcinoma fell by 42% between 1988 and 1997, with 2221 new cases registered in 2004 (the most recent year for which figures are available), and the incidence continues to fall. It is now estimated that 80% of cases are prevented by the CSP. There were 889 deaths in England in 2004 due to cervical cancer (Figures 1.1 and 1.2).

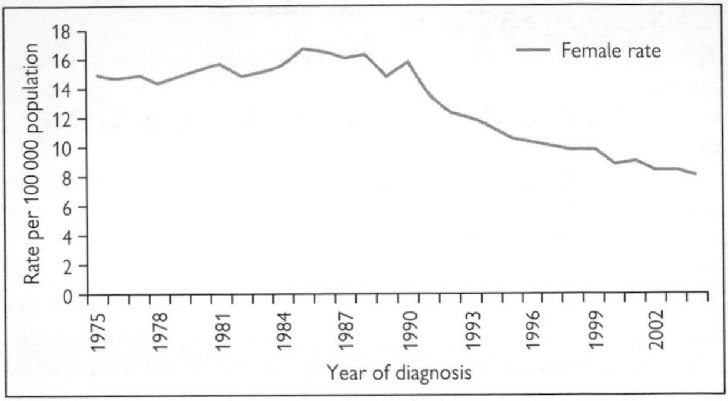

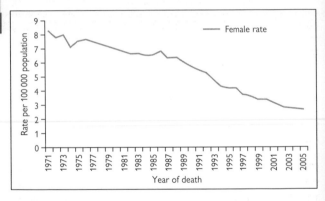

Figure 1.1 UK cervical cancer incidence (Cancer Research, UK). Cancer Research UK, www.cancerresearch.org.uk, accessed October 2007.

Age standardized (European) incidence rates, cervical cancer, GB, 1975–2004.

Figure 1.2 UK cervical cancer mortality (Cancer Research, UK). Cancer Research UK, www.cancerresearch.org.uk, accessed October 2007.

Age standardized (European) mortality rates, cervical cancer, UK, 1971–2005.

1.2 Defining features of cervical screening in the United Kingdom

The NHS CSP is a fully integrated programme, extending across the screening age range and connecting all the professional disciplines involved. This distinguishes it from many other countries, where each clinical interaction stands alone. In England, screening commences at 25 years and continues until 64, every 3 years until 50, and every 5 years thereafter. In the other developed administrations, screening begins at 20 years.

1.2.1 **Screening population**

High population coverage is essential for effective cervical screening. Cervical cancer is predominantly a disease of the less affluent; even without invitation, affluent women are more likely to present themselves for screening.

The United Kingdom has a population database, which includes all women registered with an NHS general practitioner (GP), and which is essential to run the CSP. When women register, their details are sent to a central computer database, known as the Exeter system. Data on screening can be added to and accessed from any part of the country.

This is so essential to the functioning of the CSP that a special exemption from legislation on data protection has been granted, allowing free transfer of electronic data without specific consent.

1.2.2 **Call/recall offices**

The Exeter system is delivered through call/recall offices, which are under the control of primary care trusts (PCTs). Their role is to generate lists of women due for a first call or recall. Many offices send out letters of invitation on behalf of the programme, though this task is occasionally performed by the GP. The call/recall office also has roles associated with failsafe (see Section 1.6).

1.2.3 **Terminology and standard management**

All cervical cytology in the United Kingdom is reported using the British Society of Cervical Cytology (BSCC) classification. The Bethesda System is widely used internationally, and the two systems can be roughly translated, though there are subtle differences (Table 1.1).

The cytology report differs from those produced in some other countries in that it also includes a management instruction, and these are nationally standardized.

1.2.4 **Sample takers**

The majority of UK sample takers are nurses, working in general practice. All sample takers must undergo training which includes not only the method of taking a sample but also a full understanding of the CSP. The entire clinical interaction for most women will be with this sample taker, so training must ensure a full understanding of the programme to enable accurate information to be given.

1.3 **Cytology laboratories**

Cytology laboratories are a high profile part of the NHS and are subject to very tight standards and quality assurance. All samples must be reported using Liquid-Based Cytology (LBC) by September 2008. Currently there are two manufacturers' systems; ThinPrep® (Cytyc) and SurePath® (TriPath imaging) approved for use in the United Kingdom. Cytology laboratories receive the samples, process, and report them. All samples are screened and then reviewed by a second screener. Screening is a highly skilled and painstaking process. Abnormal samples are seen by a pathologist, or more recently an advanced biomedical scientist practitioner, an extended role that allows such highly trained individuals to report abnormal cytology. Laboratories produce reports and operate a failsafe protocol for abnormal samples, as well as report positive predictive values for CIN2 or greater for high grade cytology; this is expected to be at least 65% (Table 1.2).

Table 1.1 Cervical cytology

BSCC Classification (1986)	The Bethesda System
Inadequate	Unsatisfactory for evaluation
Negative	Negative for intraepithelial lesion or malignancy
Borderline change	Atypical squamous cells of undetermined significance (ASCUS)
Mild dyskaryosis	Low-grade squamous intraepithelial lesion (LSIL)
Moderate dyskaryosis / Severe dyskaryosis	High-grade squamous intra epithelial lesion (HSIL)
Severe dyskaryosis? Invasive	Squamous cell carcinoma
?Glandular neoplasia	Atypical glandular cells

Source: http://www.blackwellpublishing.com/journal.asp?ref=0956-5507&site=1

Table 1.2 Management of abnormal cytology

Borderline change 1st occurrence	Repeat 6 months
Borderline change 2nd occurrence	Repeat 6 months or refer
Borderline change 3rd occurrence	Refer to colposcopy
Mild dyskaryosis 1st occurrence	Ideally refer to colposcopy
Mild dyskaryosis 2nd occurrence	Refer to colposcopy
Third low grade in 10 years	Refer to colposcopy
Moderate or severe dyskaryosis	Refer to colposcopy
Severe dyskaryosis? Invasive?	Urgent colposcopy referral
?Glandular neoplasia	Urgent colposcopy referral

1.4 **Colposcopy**

Most colposcopy referrals are a result of abnormal cytology. Women with symptoms such as abnormal bleeding should be referred by their GP to a gynaecologist regardless of findings on cytology, which is consequently not recommended in this setting. Many areas have implemented direct referral from the laboratory to the colposcopy clinic, which has advantages in failsafe and in shortening waiting time.

1.5 **Histopathology**

Colposcopy generates both small, diagnostic biopsies and excision specimens. These are all reported according to agreed criteria. Biopsies, which do not correlate with the referral cytology, are identified and will usually be discussed at a correlation or mismatch meeting. Reasons for lack of correlation include cytology overcall, histology undercall, and clinical issues, such as a biopsy taken from the wrong area. Lesions high in the canal, both glandular and squamous are, in particular, likely to cause a problem. This meeting provides a setting in which the woman's future management can be agreed.

In the event of a diagnosis of cervical cancer, a woman is no longer part of the screening programme; however, links to oncology services are obviously important.

1.6 **Failsafe**

A feature of the NHS CSP, and of all successful screening programmes, is failsafe. This is the process by which women who have not progressed through the required processes of screening at any stage are identified, so that action can be taken to rectify the situation. This means that action is taken to remind women who do not attend for a smear when invited; and for women with abnormal smears, failsafe processes check that they have been referred for colposcopy, and attended to. All parts of the CSP are involved in interlinked failsafe processes. Inevitably, some women will decide not to participate in the programme, even after they have had an abnormal sample, and there are agreed endpoints for such women in terms of failsafe, though they may re-enter the programme at any point.

1.7 **Management of the programme**

In England, cervical screening is commissioned by PCTs for their population, often in shared, lead purchaser agreements. A key individual is the screening commissioner, usually a public health professional, who is responsible for specifying and monitoring the local programme, including the parts such as sample taking, call and recall, and failsafe, which are provided by the PCT or staff in primary care. Most of the services are provided by acute trusts, and the key management role here is that of the hospital-based programme coordinator. This will be a senior member of staff who monitors the performance of the trust in pathology and colposcopy, and works closely with the screening commissioner to ensure that specifications are being met.

1.8 Quality assurance

All aspects of the NHS CSP are subject to rigorous quality assurance, based on a raft of publications which define the minimum requirements for the service (NHS CSP Publications www.cancerscreening.nhs.uk). These are evolving documents that are based on published evidence, accepted practice, and comparison with other screening programmes. All parts of the programme are monitored with defined statistical returns which are published by the Department of Health, and for some measures, for example, the detection rate for abnormalities, 10th–90th centiles are used to identify outliers which require further investigation. This is one of the functions of the quality assurance teams (QATs), regionally based teams of professionals from all parts of the programme, who visit, monitor, and advise, as well as identify and publicize good practice. The QATs are also responsible for administering external quality assurance schemes for cytology reporting and technical slide preparation. The cornerstone of internal quality assurance is a rapid review of all samples—meaning that all negatives are reviewed by two members of staff. Abnormalities missed on the first screen are recorded, and screeners must maintain 95% sensitivity for high-grade abnormalities and 90% for all grades. Failure to do so results in monitoring and possible retraining, and ultimately, if persistent, the screener may be redeployed to another role.

From May 2001, it has been mandatory for all cases of cervical cancer to be audited, with the result being offered to the women. Devising an agreed protocol was difficult, but the protocol was implemented in April 2007. The process is administered by the QATs. The purpose of the audit is entirely educational, though it remains to be seen whether such audit and disclosure results in increased litigation.

Well-publicized deficiencies in screening programme quality in the past, especially incidents at Kent and Canterbury in 1996, have resulted in quality assurance having a central place in the NHS CSP.

1.8.1 The NHS CSP

The whole programme is overseen by a national programme director who is responsible for development of all national policies, and reports at a high level within the Department of Health. This role has been critical to the development of the CSP. The Department of Health receives advice on the programme from a multiprofessional advisory committee.

1.9 Future developments

Apart from human papilloma virus (HPV) testing and vaccination, there are a number of other developments which may impact on screening. Both manufactures of LBC, currently working within the United Kingdom, have automated systems which in studies elsewhere maintain screening accuracy while greatly increasing productivity. These systems are currently being tested in a complex trial manual versus automated reading in cytology (MAVARIC) whose outcome is expected in 2010. If successful, this will have major implications for organization of cytology services.

Perhaps more distantly there are a number of other possible developments in biomarkers, some with semi-automated reading. These include immunohistochemical methods for p16 and various proliferation markers. None of these is yet ready to test in a UK screening environment.

1.10 Problems faced by the UK CSPs

The CSP has been very successful at reducing the incidence of cervical cancer, but there is still room for improvement. Each year, around 4 million women have a cervical cytology sample in England and Wales, and even with LBC, around 7% receive a result that is not negative. The majority of these have low-grade abnormalities, and then embark on a period of cytology surveillance or referral which is stressful. Yet only around 2000 women per year are diagnosed with cervical cancer, so clearly there is an issue that specificity of the test could be improved. Conversely women still develop cervical cancer after having been fully screened—showing that the sensitivity of the test could also be improved.

Testing for HPV has been proposed as a potential solution to both these issues.

Possible models of introducing HPV into the CSP are as follows:

• HPV as primary screening.
• HPV testing for triage of low grade abnormalities (see Chapters 5 and 11).

1.11 **The cervical screening programme, threats, and challenges**

There is no doubt that the CSP has been successful, but as it matures it does face threats.

Falling population coverage, especially in younger women. There is persistent evidence of falling coverage, especially in women in the 25–29 age group. Reasons for this are not known, but may include general features of this age group reflected in low rates of other community-based activities. The success of the CSP is probably a factor—nowadays few women know someone who has had cervical cancer. Combating this complacency is a challenge for primary care. Improving access for women of all cultures is important, as well as the quality of written information. Recently, several programmes have launched advertisements with eye-catching slogans, backed up by radio and television articles to try to reach this group of women.

Publicity. In the past, the CSP has been the subject of very negative publicity, but the balance now appears to be restored. There is a growing understanding that cytology interpretation is an opinion, and is thus subject to inconsistency and error, which may not be negligible. Publicity has been very positive over such issues as the implementation of LBC, and the recent announcement—that all women will receive their result in 2 weeks—carried welcome positive publicity with it, though this will be a challenge to implement.

Maintaining a skilled workforce. Cervical cytology requires a highly trained and skilled workforce. The advent of LBC, HPV testing, and extended roles for biomedical scientists is attracting very high calibre applicants, but many laboratories still find it hard to appoint staff. Since services are reconfigured, staff may not wish to move, and this could be a problem. Implementation of technologies which reduce the number of abnormal smears will make maintaining individual staff exposure to abnormalities difficult. Staffing problems have been improved by the implementation of LBC with its improvements in productivity.

Service reconfigurations and maintaining integrity of the programme in the face of increased diversity of providers within the NHS. The government commissioned Lord Carter to report on provision of pathology within the NHS. Cervical cytology was not a major focus to this report but there are implications. Service reconfiguration seems inevitable and is welcome in many ways, but care will be needed to ensure that multidisciplinary clinical links are not compromised.

Novel screening and prevention modalities. Novel screening modalities do not in themselves represent a threat to cervical screening. If they are implemented, it will be after a rigorous evaluation so that their costs and effectiveness in the UK setting are known. There are challenges, ranging from education of the public, through reconfigurations, staff changes, and maintaining expertise that will need to be met. A key fact is that expertise in administering a screening programme and knowledge of cervical cytology are currently vested in the same individuals. If modalities change, it will be critical to maintain this expertise within such a programme. There is also a challenge to ensure that women realize that new modalities do not mean that they no longer need to attend for screening, and this is particularly an issue with the HPV vaccine.

1.12 **Conclusion**

The CSP has been continuing in a low profile way for many years, but the last 15 years have seen huge developments in all aspects of screening programme management. The next phase will be the introduction of new techniques into this rapidly evolving area. Cervical cancer is already a rare condition and will continue to decline. This represents the ultimate success for cervical screening in the United Kingdom.

11

Further reading

Denton KJ (2007). Liquid based cytology for cervical screening. In James Underwood, Massimo Pignatelli, eds. *Recent advances in histopathology*, 22pp. Royal Society of Medicine Press, London.

Moss SM, Gray A, Marteau T, Legood R, Henstock E, Maissi E (2004). Evaluation of HPV/LBC Cervical screening pilot studies. Report to the Department of Health 2004. www.cancerscreening.nhs.uk/cervical/evaluation-hpv-2006feb.pdf

NHS CSP publications. Cervical Screening reviews 2005 and 2006 NHS CSP publications 1–29. www.cancerscreening.nhs.uk.

Peto J, Gilham C, Fletcher O, Mathews FE (2004). The cervical screening epidemic that screening has prevented in the UK. *Lancet*, **364**: 249–56.

Raffle AE and Muir Gray JA (2007). *Screening: evidence and practice*. Oxford University Press, Oxford.

Report of the Review of Pathology services in England. Lord Carter of Coles. Department of Health. www.dh.gov.uk/publications.

Chapter 2

Management of cervical intraepithelial neoplasia (CIN)

Julia E Palmer and John A Tidy

Key points

- CIN is a relatively common problem.
- CIN1 may be managed conservatively in appropriate circumstances.
- CIN2/3 should be treated.
- Excisional or ablative treatments are available.
- Patients should be counselled and techniques used appropriate to individual situations.
- Overall treatments are >90% effective.
- Women diagnosed with CIN remain at risk of recurrent or persistent CIN and the development of cervical carcinoma.
- Follow-up is essential.

2.1 Introduction

Cervical cancer registrations and deaths from disease have continued to decline in the United Kingdom since the advent of the NHS cervical screening programme. Approximately 4 million women are invited for screening each year, with approximately 3.5 million women subsequently attending. Between 2006 and 2007, there were 118 600 first attendances at colposcopy out of a total of almost 400 000 appointments: 40% were appointments for a first visit, 8% were for treatment, and 52% were for some form of follow-up. Approximately 46 000 biopsies were taken in this time period. Excisional biopsies performed for treatment of colposcopic abnormalities revealed evidence of CIN2 or worse in 67% of cases.

CIN is, therefore, a very common disease, especially in women of reproductive age, and a balance needs to maximize the prevention of cervical carcinoma and at the same time avoid over treatment.

Management strategies of CIN include decision-making regarding the appropriateness of a conservative approach versus treatment. Conservative strategies are appropriate for women with low-grade CIN, particularly in the younger age range. High-grade CIN (CIN2 or worse) should be treated. Conservative methods reduce over-treatment as low-grade CIN lesions may spontaneously regress. Conservative management, however, requires accurate colposcopic assessment, confirmation of low-grade CIN by directed biopsy, and adherence to follow-up.

2.2 Diagnosis of CIN

Women referred with an abnormal cytology result should undergo colposcopic examination. Colposcopy permits assessment of the transformation zone for the presence of CIN and the accurate targeting of biopsy. The clinical assessment of CIN (colposcopic impression) has a positive predictive value (PPV) of 65–85% for high-grade CIN and 50–60% for low-grade CIN, which is similar to that of cytology. The diagnosis of CIN requires either a punch biopsy or a loop cone biopsy.

In cases where low-grade CIN (CIN1) is confirmed either by colposcopic impression or by directed biopsy, conservative management is recommended. In many young women a low-grade abnormality is probably a reflection simply of human papilloma virus infection. Cytology and colposcopy should be performed 6–12 monthly and if the low-grade abnormality persists, then repeat biopsy at least, is recommended within 2 years of follow-up. Treatment should be considered and will often be requested by women if the low-grade abnormality persists for longer than 24 months.

2.3 Indications for treatment

When high-grade CIN (CIN2 or worse) is diagnosed, treatment is mandatory. CIN3, which is the true precursor of cancer, will progress to cancer if untreated at a rate of around 30% over 20 years. For adenocarcinoma, the precursor lesion is cervical glandular intraepithelial neoplasia.

CIN1 has been reported to progress to CIN2/3 at a rate of 15% over 2 years, but some of these cases may harbour undetected CIN2/3.

2.4 **Treatment policies**

Variation in treatment patterns may occur in both those attending with high- and low-grade CIN, and at local and regional levels. A 'see and treat' policy means offering women who are thought to have high-grade CIN, immediate lesion excision using large loop excision transformation zone (LLETZ). The advantages of a 'see and treat' policy are that at-risk patients are treated and occult cancers are detected without delay. Early experience with this method of management led to over-treatment. A 'select and treat' policy of offering treatment at first visit to women referred with moderate or severe dyskaryosis is now recommended to reduce the risk of over-treatment of women who turn out not to have CIN. Deferred treatment is advantageous in that it reduces over-treatment, yet it is a less efficient use of resources, increasing the burden of both counselling and follow-up. It should be noted that almost 20% of excisional biopsies were reported showing no CIN, suggesting that there is further scope to avoid over-treatment from needless excision.

2.5 **Treatment techniques**

The two main methods of treatment are ablative and excisional (see Table 2.1). Excisional techniques allow comprehensive histological investigation of the tissue and the entire transformation zone, with precise assessment of excision margins. Excisional techniques enable the implementation of a 'see and treat' policy at the primary visit. Conversely, ablative techniques destroy the transformation zone epithelium, thus precluding histological diagnosis. Therefore, before treatment, colposcopically directed biopsy samples must be taken at a separate primary visit. Both techniques, however, have reported cure rates of over 90%.

All treatments should be performed with adequate anaesthesia. Treatment should be offered with local analgesia, but general anaesthesia should be offered if a woman either cannot tolerate a procedure under local anaesthetic or is adamant that she will not agree to local anaesthesia.

Ablative techniques should only be performed when colposcopy and directed biopsy have excluded invasion. Ablative techniques are suitable when

- The transformation zone is visualized in its entirety.
- There is no evidence of glandular abnormality.
- There is no evidence of invasive disease.
- There is no major discrepancy between cytology and histology.

Table 2.1 Excisional and ablative techniques	
Excisional techniques	**Ablative techniques**
Large loop excision transformation zone (LLETZ)/Loop electrosurgical excision procedure (LEEP)	Laser ablation
Laser excision of TZ/laser conization	Cryocautery
Loop/cold knife cone biopsy	Cold coagulation
Hysterectomy	Radical/electrodiathermy

2.5.1 Laser ablation

Laser ablation uses a CO_2 laser and will accurately ablate the transformation zone in terms of both depth (usually 7–10mm) and width. Laser ablation is advantageous in that it causes minimal damage to adjacent structures, can be used to treat extended vaginal lesions, and has few side effects. Cure rates of between 90% and 95% can be expected following treatment of CIN.

2.5.2 Cryocautery

Cryocautery utilizes either an N_2O or CO_2 probe and freezes the cervix to $-70°C$ to $-90°C$. A 2-minute treatment is required for a 5mm depth of penetration. Larger lesions may require multiple applications. Cryocautery is advantageous in that it is 'low-tech', of relatively low cost, does not require analgesia, and has low complication rates, but its disadvantage is the generally poor depth of penetration attained. Cryocautery results in approximately 4–6% and 10–38% treatment failures for CIN1/2 and CIN3, respectively, with treatment failure rates also increasing with larger lesions. This technique is not recommended because of unacceptably high treatment failure rates, and should only be used for low-grade CIN. A double freeze–thaw–freeze technique has a lower incidence of residual disease compared with a single freeze technique. Because it is a 'low-tech' method, its use has been considered following a positive visual inspection aided by acetic acid (VIA) in resource poor settings.

2.5.3 Cold coagulation

Cold coagulation utilizes heat (50–120°C) to destroy tissue, with the depth of tissue penetration exceeding 4mm when performed at higher temperatures. It is advantageous in that it is a relatively cost-efficient procedure, requiring no analgesia, having few complications and good cure rates, but measurement of depth of tissue destruction is difficult.

2.5.4 Electrodiathermy

Electrodiathermy uses either a ball or a needlepoint set at 40–50 Watts coagulation to ablate tissue. Approximately 7mm depth of tissue penetration can be achieved, providing excellent cure rates irrespective of grade of CIN. Similar to other ablative techniques, electrodiathermy has few complications and is a simple, fast, and cost-effective technique to perform. It is not widely used now because it has a greater need for general anaesthesia (see Table 2.2).

2.6 Excisional treatment techniques

For ectocervical lesions, excisional techniques should remove tissue to a depth of 7mm because of the depth of crypt involvement by CIN3. For endocervical lesions, incomplete excision at the endocervical margin requires repeat colposcopy and cytology at 6 months after treatment. Further excision is recommended if there is residual CIN on biopsy or positive high-grade dyskaryosis because up to 15% of patients with incomplete excisions will develop recurrent cytological abnormalities. For women over 50 years, consideration should be given to routine repeat excision for involved margins because of the high rate of residual CIN. Excisional techniques should generally remove the specimen as a single sample in the majority of cases because fragmentation can cause difficulty in histopathological assessment, and if microinvasive disease is present allocation of a sub-stage or assessment of completeness of excision is impossible.

2.6.1 Large loop excision of the transformation zone (LLETZ)

The most common excisional technique, LLETZ, enables excision of the entire transformation zone using single-pass or multiple-pass techniques in larger lesions. Loop size is chosen according to the

Table 2.2 Complications of ablative techniques

	Immediate	Short term	Long term	Cure rate %
Laser ablation	Pain	Few	Few	>90
Cryocautery	Pain <1% 1° haemorrhage (1%)	• 2° haemorrhage (1–2%) • Infection • Vaginal discharge	Cervical stenosis (1–2%)	60–90
Cold coagulation	Pain	• Vaginal discharge • Vaginal bleeding (up to 6 weeks)	Few	94
Electrodiathermy	Few	• 2° haemorrhage (1–2%)	Fibrosis	98

lesion size and size of TZ. The technique may be performed using a straight wire. LLETZ is an inexpensive, quick, and relatively easy process, which can be used in a 'see and treat' setting. Cure rates are high (94–98%), but without careful selection it can result in over-treatment.

2.6.2 Laser conization

Laser conization is performed using CO_2 or an Nd:YAG laser. Laser techniques allow good control of tissue depth penetration with less thermal damaged margins than LLETZ, and have reported cure rates of 95%. The technique is disadvantageous in that it takes longer to perform and the equipment is expensive.

2.6.3 Knife cone biopsy

Knife cone biopsy is generally to confirm invasive disease, to excise endocervical CIN, and to diagnose glandular lesions. A scalpel is used and general anaesthesia is required. Knife cone biopsy, however, has an increased risk of haemorrhage and ensuing cervical stenosis. Cure rates are lower than using the techniques described above because therapeutic knife cone is reserved for women with endocervical disease.

2.7 Hysterectomy

Hysterectomy is a recognized treatment for histologically proven CIN if significant coexisting gynaecological conditions are present that render such surgery appropriate. Hysterectomy is also acceptable for persistent abnormal endocervical cytology following unsuccessful conservative treatment. Hysterectomy should only be performed as a treatment for CIN when occult invasion has been excluded. Simple hysterectomy may be considered when

- Fertility is not required.
- Positive endocervical margins remain following an excisional procedure for endocervical disease.
- Further high-grade cytological abnormality occurs following treatment by cone biopsy, in the absence of upper vaginal disease.
- Microinvasive disease.
- Patients have other clinical indications for surgery.
- Patients are unwilling to undergo conservative management.

A colposcopic examination should be performed immediately prior to hysterectomy to ensure that the entire lesion and transformation zone will be excised. Cure rates from hysterectomy are >95%, but follow-up may be required depending on histological findings, particularly if CIN was present in the hysterectomy specimen.

2.8 **Summary**

Meta-analysis has shown no obvious superior technique for the treatment of CIN (Table 2.3). Excisional techniques, however, are reported to result in lower rates of moderately dyskaryotic smears following treatment, as compared with ablative techniques.

2.9 **Management of cervical glandular intraepithelial neoplasia (CGIN)**

Management of CGIN differs somewhat from the management of CIN. Colposcopic impression and punch biopsy are regarded as unreliable in the diagnosis of CGIN, which is associated with high levels of both pre-invasive and invasive disease. CGIN should be managed using excisional techniques to ensure that adequate margins of excision are attained and the use of knife cone biopsy is supported. A cylindrical knife cone up to 25mm in depth will suffice in most cases. If margins of excision are incomplete then repeat excision should be considered. For women wishing to retain their fertility, a further cone biopsy may be considered, but hysterectomy is appropriate when preserving fertility is not important.

2.10 **Obstetric outcomes following treatment for CIN and CGIN**

Available evidence suggests that fertility is not impaired after treatment for CIN. Meta-analysis has reported knife cone biopsy to be associated with an increased risk of pre-term labour, low birth-weight,

Table 2.3 Cochrane Review findings	
Ablative treatments	**Excisional treatments**
Double freezing techniques more successful than single freezing	Laser versus Knife Cone Biopsy • No difference found in residual disease • Laser has less cervical stenosis and unsatisfactory colposcopy at follow-up, but more artefact damage
In comparision to cryocautery, laser ablation has more post-treatment bleeding	Laser versus LLETZ • LLETZ quicker to perform. Laser greater artefact damage
With the exception of cryocautery, cure rates are similar	Knife Cone versus LLETZ • Knife cone has less residual disease • Knife cone has lower unsatisfactory colposcopy rates at follow-up

and caesarean section. LLETZ was also found to be associated with pre-term labour, low birth-weight, and premature rupture of the membranes, particularly if the depth of the excised specimen is greater than one centimetre. These findings, as yet, have failed to identify reliable groups of women at increased risk of an adverse obstetric outcome; such groups may include those who undergo extensive diathermy and large or repeated excisions. Caution is therefore recommended in the treatment of young women with low-grade lesions, and attention should be paid to avoiding excessively and unnecessary deep excisions, particularly when colposcopy is satisfactory.

2.11 **Patient counselling**

Patients undergoing treatment for CIN should be thoroughly counselled, including advice regarding the nature of their treatment, available anaesthetic techniques, and cure rates. Post-operative advice regarding the likelihood of vaginal discharge and bleeding and avoidance of tampons and intercourse for 4 weeks post-treatment should also be given with contact numbers provided.

2.12 **Follow-up**

Women treated for CIN remain at risk of persistent or recurrent CIN and the development of cervical carcinoma. The risk of cancer has been estimated at 1 in 200 over 8 years of follow-up. Follow-up is therefore essential and up until now has relied on annual cytology over 10 years.

For conservatively managed low-grade lesions, 6–12 monthly follow-up cytology and colposcopy should be performed, and if the low-grade abnormality persists then repeat biopsy at least is recommended within 2 years of follow-up.

Treatment failures most commonly occur within the first 2 years. Treatment failure rates should not exceed 10% and in many centres is not more than 5%. Recurrence of CIN is more common following positive excision margins, particularly if the endocervical margin was incompletely excised. Cytological follow-up is, therefore, most frequently performed in the first 2 years after treatment.

Women treated for CGIN are at a higher risk of developing recurrent disease than those with high-grade CIN, thus cytological follow-up is performed more frequently than in CIN. Cytological follow-up should be offered to all treated patients and colposcopy performed when cytological abnormality is detected (see Figure 2.1).

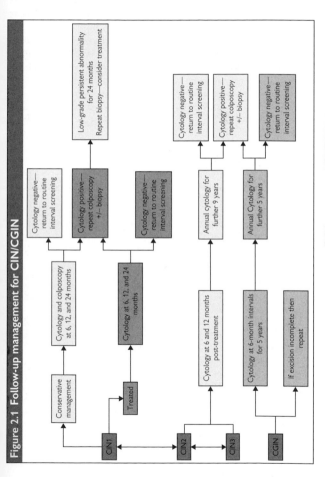

Figure 2.1 Follow-up management for CIN/CGIN

Following hysterectomy, women with CIN are at risk of vaginal intraepithelial neoplasia (VAIN). If CIN was noted at hysterectomy, though fully excised, current recommendations advise vault smears at 6 and 18 months post-operatively then discontinuation of follow-up if cytology is normal. If margins are incompletely excised, however, or doubt exists as to the completeness of excision, then these patients should be followed up as if the cervix remains in-situ.

Human papilloma virus (HPV) testing for post-treatment follow-up is reported to out-perform cytological follow-up in the detection of persistent/recurrent CIN. HPV testing has a very high negative predictive value, potentially allowing rapid return to routine recall if cytology and HPV are both negative at 6 months. This has been confirmed in a recent UK study of 900 treated women. HPV as test of cure has now been incorporated in a pilot study for the NHS CSP (see Chapters 5 and 11).

Suggested reading

Cervical screening program 2005–2006. The information centre. ISBN: 1-84636-095-1; Bulletin: 2006/24/HSCIC.

Kitchener HC, Walker PG, Nelson L, Hadwin R, Patnick J, Anthony GB, Sargent A, Wood J, Moore C, Cruickshank M (2008). HPV testing as an adjunct to cytology in the follow-up of women treated for cervical intraepithelial neoplasia. *British Journal of Obstetrics and Gynaecology*, **115**; 1001–7.

Kyrgiou M, Koliopoulos G, Martin-Hirsch P, Arbyn M, Preddiville, W, Paraskevaidis, E (2006). Obstetric outcomes after conservative treatment for intraepithelial or early invasive cervical lesions: systematic review and meta-analysis. *Lancet,* **367**: 489–98.

Leusley DM, Leeson S (2004). Colposcopy and programme management: guidelines for the NHS cervical screening programme. NHSCSP publication No 20. Sheffield: NHSCSP Publications, April 2004.

Martin-Hirsch P, Paraskevaidis E, Kitchener, HC (2000). Surgery for cervical intraepithelial neoplasia. *Cochrane Database System Review,* **2**, CD001318.

Wright TC, Jr., Massad LS, Dunton, CJ, Spitzer M, Wilkinson EJ, Solomon D. (2007). 2006 consensus guidelines for the management of women with cervical intraepithelial neoplasia or adenocarcinoma *in situ. American Journal of Obstetrics and Gynecology*, **197**: 340–5.

Part 2

HPV and disease

Chapter 3

Role of HPV in cervical carcinogenesis

Sally Roberts and Lawrence S Young

Key points

- Infection of squamous epithelia by specific human papilloma virus (HPV) types contributes to the development of cervical cancer; HPV 16 and HPV 18 are the most common oncogenic types present in cervical carcinomas.
- The E6 and E7 oncoproteins, by dysregulating host cell cycle control and abrogating the host cell's anti-proliferative response, promote the proliferation and survival of HPV infected cells.
- Persistent expression of E6 and E7 oncoproteins allow the accumulation of genetic mutations that can lead to cellular immortalization and finally malignant conversion.
- Integration of the HPV genome into the host chromosome, a common event in high-grade CIN and cervical carcinomas, up-regulates expression of E6 and E7 oncoproteins.
- Cervical cancer is a late and rare complication of a persistent HPV infection and is the end result of a chain of events that can take many years to unfold—infection with HPV is necessary but not a sufficient cause of cervical cancer.

3.1 The virus

3.1.1 Multiple HPV types

Human papilloma viruses (HPVs) infect epithelial tissues (e.g. skin, mucosa) at many different body sites, gaining entry through minor cuts and abrasions, and frequently inducing benign growths known as warts or papillomas. In most instances, the infection does not elicit any serious clinical problem and the papillomas eventually regress, but some infections can occasionally persist and progress to cancer.

HPVs are classified into groups or species according to the sequence of their genome, and so far, in excess of 100 types have been identified. Only a small number of HPV types inflict infections that have the potential to proceed to a malignancy (Table 3.1). Of the 15 HPV types that are deemed to be high risk in the development of anogenital cancer, HPV 16 and HPV 18 have the greatest oncogenic risk, accounting for nearly 70% of all cervical cancers. In squamous cell carcinoma of the cervix, HPV 16 is the most frequent type (over 50% of cancers) followed by HPV 18 (between 15% and 20% of cancers), whereas HPV 18 is the type most strongly associated with cervical adenocarcinoma (ADC). Some of these anogenital high-risk viruses have also been linked to the aetiology of cancers that arise in the oropharynx. At the other end of the scale are types such as HPV 6 and HPV 11, that are termed low-risk viruses because they are only rarely associated with cancers (Table 3.1). Despite their lower oncogenic potential, these viruses are most commonly associated with benign genital warts (condylomas) and laryngeal papillomas that are in themselves a significant clinical burden to the human population.

A significant number of HPV types also show a tropism for the skin or cutaneous epithelia, at body sites other than the anogenital region. Most of these cutaneous types induce benign warts, for example, common hand warts caused by HPV 1, but some (e.g. types 8 and 38) are associated with non-melanoma skin cancers (Table 3.1). The study of these HPV types has highlighted the importance of the host immune recognition system in controlling infections by HPV, as these high-risk cutaneous types are especially prevalent in immunocompromised individuals such as organ transplant recipients.

3.1.2 **HPV structure**

HPV is a small virus of 55nm diameter and comprises a double-stranded circular DNA of nearly 8000 base pairs (Figure 3.1). The coat of the virus is made up of two proteins, the major one being L1 and a

HPV type	Site of infection	Associated lesion	Oncogenic risk
1, 4	Cutaneous skin	Common hand warts, verrucae	Benign
6, 11	Anogenital epithelia and laryngeal mucosa	Genital warts, laryngeal papillomas	Low
16, 18, 33, 45	Anogenital epithelia and oropharyngeal mucosa	CIN, anogenital cancers including cervical carcinoma, oropharyngeal cancer	High
5, 8, 38	Cutaneous skin	Non-melanoma skin cancer	High

Table 3.1 **Examples of HPV types, their infection site, associated disease, and oncogenic potential**

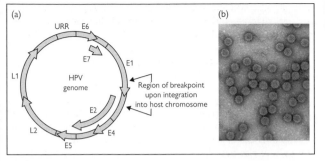

Figure 3.1 Structure of HPV: (a) Organization of HPV double-stranded genome. (b) Electron micrograph of HPV virions. Image reproduced courtesy of B Garcea, University of Colorado Health Sciences, USA.

minor component L2. The coat proteins assemble into structures known as capsomeres and 72 of these come together to form the spherical coat. The ability of L1 when expressed in the absence of L2 to assemble spontaneously into particles that appear to be very similar to the native virions has been the major driving force behind the development of HPV prophylactic vaccines. The HPV genome encodes eight proteins:

- Early proteins E5, E6, and E7 are involved in cell proliferation and survival, and E6 and E7 play a key role in HPV-associated carcinogenesis.
- Three other early proteins (E1, E2, and E4) are involved in control of viral gene transcription and viral DNA replication.
- Two late proteins L1 and L2 are involved in the assembly of new virus particles.

3.2 **HPV replication in the host**

3.2.1 **The HPV life cycle**

In an HPV infection, the sole aim of the virus is to replicate itself to produce progeny infectious virions. Cancer may result when the process of replication is inhibited in some way. This aborted infection is of no benefit to the virus as the host cell is no longer permissive for virion production. In a normal infection, the virus replication cycle is inextricably linked to the life history of the host epithelial cell (Figure 3.2). However, HPV is not a passive passenger in this process, but one that re-programmes the cell to permit its own replication and the production of large numbers of new infectious virions.

The virus enters cells within the basal layer of the epithelium, whereupon the genome is uncoated and transferred to the cell's nucleus where it exists as a non-integrated circular episome of less than 100 copies per cell. As these infected basal cells undergo cell division, the viral genome replicates and becomes equally segregated between the two daughter cells, enabling maintenance of the HPV genome in this cell layer. New virus production, however, is inhibited in these cells and the process of a productive infection only begins once the infected basal cell begins its migration upwards into the above layers—the suprabasal layers. In an uninfected epithelium, the upward migration of basal cells triggers their exit from the cell cycle and they enter the pathway of terminal differentiation. Because HPV relies heavily on the host cell for provision of key replication enzymes and other factors necessary to replicate its own genome, the loss of this machinery in suprabasal cells poses a serious problem for the virus that needs to be overcome if it is to successfully produce new virus. The actions of the two early proteins E6 and E7 provide the answer, by stimulating the proliferation of the infected suprabasal cells (and therefore production of the cell's replication machinery) and ensuring their survival long enough for the virus to replicate its own genome (Figure 3.2). Once the virus has amplified its genome, sometimes to levels exceeding many thousands of copies per cell, the HPV life cycle then switches to production of the coat proteins L1 and L2. This stage is most likely controlled by the early E2 protein that can down-regulate the expression of the E6 and E7 proteins, by blocking the binding of transcription factors to the early virus promoter. The reduction in E6 and E7 expression removes the stimulus to retain the replication competent status and the cell completes the process of terminal differentiation. New virions are now assembled, followed by their eventual release from the uppermost cells of the squamous epithelial lesion (Figure 3.2).

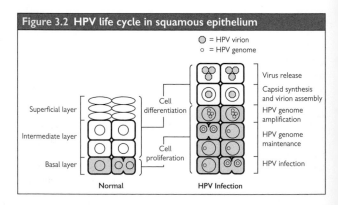

Figure 3.2 HPV life cycle in squamous epithelium

3.2.2 **Functions of E6 and E7 proteins to promote cell proliferation and survival**

The growth of cells is divided into a number of phases that make up the cell cycle. In the S phase the cellular genome is replicated to produce two exact copies, and mitotic division of the cell into two daughter cells occurs in M phase. The S and M phases are separated by gap phases (G1 and G2) (Figure 3.3). Progression from one phase to another is tightly regulated by a complex network of proteins and ensures that DNA replication and cell division occurs only if cell growth conditions are favourable. The retinoblastoma (Rb) protein is of critical importance in the control of cell proliferation, since it regulates the activity of a number of transcription factors (e.g. E2F) that trigger the expression of proteins necessary for progression of cells from G1 into S phase and replication of the cellular genome. The decision of whether the cell should proceed with genome replication is dependent on the phosphorylation state of Rb (Figure 3.3). If cell growth conditions are favourable, hyperphosphorylation of Rb takes place and E2F is released to activate expression of the proteins that drive the cell cycle into S phase. When conditions are not favourable, Rb remains in a hypophosphorylated state and E2F remains tightly bound to Rb, and as a consequence, replication of the genome does not happen.

HPV-infected cells are driven into S phase regardless of the nature of the growth conditions by E7 binding Rb and releasing E2F (Figure 3.3). The disruption of Rb function is further ensured by E7, which also promotes the inappropriate degradation of the Rb protein. The unscheduled activation of S phase should lead to apoptosis of the cell, but this is prevented by the action of E6 on pro-apoptotic proteins such as p53 and Bak. The E6 protein triggers the degradation of the apoptotic promoting factors by forming a complex with a cellular protein (E6-AP) to form an enzyme that can then direct p53 and Bak to the cell's protein degradation machinery (Figure 3.3).

Normal cells can also move into a state of non-proliferation known as senescence. An important signal for entry into senescence is the gradual shortening of structures found at the ends of chromosomes known as telomeres. Telomere erosion occurs as the cell divides and is part of the process of cell ageing. HPV avoids cell senescence by using E6 to activate telomerase, an enzyme that restores telomeres to a length that cannot trigger senescence.

The consequences of the cooperative actions of E6 and E7 on the host are that the dependence on cell cycle control is abolished and normal differentiation of the epithelial cell is retarded, and for the virus, access to the host's replication machinery and persistence of these proliferating cells is required until such time the virus has amplified its own genome.

30

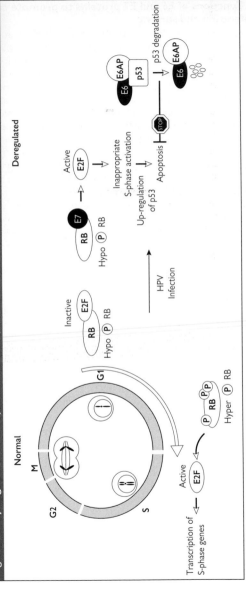

Figure 3.3 Dysregulation of cell cycle control and promotion of cell survival by E6 and E7 oncoproteins

3.3 **Oncogenic potential of HPV**

3.3.1 **Induction of genetic instability in the host**

By re-programming the epithelial cell to permit its own replication, HPV has created a cellular environment that favours increased cell proliferation and the survival of the infected cell primarily through the deregulation of two major tumour suppressor pathways. The p53 pathway also has a critical role in sensing damage to the cell's genome and enables the cell to respond to this damage either through repair of the genetic defect or by cell death (apoptosis). Inadvertently then, by abrogation of p53 function through the actions of the E6 protein, HPV allows the accumulation of secondary DNA mutations to occur and persist in the host genome; and if oncogenic mutations arise these will go unchecked, contributing to immortalization and ultimately conversion to a malignant cell. E7 function can also contribute to the genetic instability of HPV-infected cells by interfering with the normal replication of centrosomes; structures that are necessary for the faithful division of the diploid chromosome complement. Thus, in the presence of persistent expression of E6 and E7, cells frequently acquire structural chromosomal changes such as translocations, deletions, and amplification, and numerical chromosomal imbalances (aneuploidy).

3.3.2 **Integration of the HPV genome into the host chromosome**

In women with CIN1, the virus replicates in much the same way that it would in productive papillomas, where replication of the virus occurs. By the time the disease has progressed to CIN2 and CIN3, however, cells that are differentiation competent and able to support virus replication have become increasingly sparse and are most often found in restricted foci in the uppermost regions of the lesion. An important molecular change underlying CIN progression is the integration of the HPV genome into the host's genome. While integration into the host chromosome occurs at common fragile sites (site of gene transcription) that have a more or less random distribution, the site of breakage within the HPV DNA is preferentially restricted to the region covering the E1 and E2 genes with the consequence of loss of production of viral proteins other than E6 and E7 (Figure 3.1). Not only does this molecular event limit the capacity of the virus to produce progeny virions, but it also severs the negative feedback signals of the viral regulatory E2 protein on expression of E6 and E7. The result is the up-regulation of these two proteins leading to increased cell proliferation. Proof that a loss of integrity of the E2-dependent regulation of E6 and E7 expression is inextricably associated with continuous cell proliferation has been shown by the reactivation of the p53 and Rb tumour suppressor growth inhibitory pathways in cervical cancer cells following reinstatement of E2 expression.

Integration of the HPV genome, therefore, provides a growth advantage to the host cells, and the continuous uncontrolled proliferation of a cell that has already been genetically compromised increases the likelihood of the acquisition of oncogenic mutations. It is therefore of no surprise that although cells containing HPV-integrated forms can be detected in low-grade cervical disease, they become much more frequent as the disease progresses to CIN3, and in cancers themselves, greater than 70% of metastatic cells can contain HPV integrants.

3.3.3 Why are only some HPV types oncogenic?

Of the large number of HPV types found in infections of the cervix, only as few as 15 are associated with cancers (Table 3.1). There are no major differences in the structure of these viruses that could immediately explain the difference in oncogenicity. Differences only become apparent on comparison of E6 and E7 functions between high- and low-risk viruses:

- Low-risk E6 proteins do not stimulate the degradation of p53.
- The telomerase enzyme is not activated by low-risk E6 gene products.
- Low-risk E7 proteins bind Rb, but less efficiently than do high-risk proteins, and do not induce degradation of Rb.
- There is no evidence of disruption of centrosomes by low-risk E7 proteins.

3.4 Cervical cancer is a multistep disease

That HPV has a causal role in the development of cancer of the cervix is in no doubt. Some 99.7% of cervical cancers actually contain oncogenic forms of the virus. Of the estimated 291 million women who harbour an infection with a high-risk HPV, most (80%) will be transient or have persistent infections with no identifiable symptoms. Others will lead to a CIN, which may or may not then progress to cancer. Among the cervical abnormalities that develop, most early lesions will regress spontaneously but the rate of regression decreases with increasing severity of the CIN. Cervical cancer is a late and rare complication of a persistent HPV infection and is the end result of a chain of events that take, in most instances, in excess of 10 years to unfold.

Many studies have shown that the E6 and E7 proteins from high-risk types act together to immortalize the host cell, but that this is not sufficient to cause their full transformation into a tumour cell, indicating the need for additional genetic events. The virus itself sets the scene by initiating the process of genetic instability through de-regulation of various tumour suppressor pathways. If the infection persists then there is increased likelihood that mutations will be acquired that promote cell immortalization, transformation, and eventually metastasis. The situation is further exaggerated by increased production of the two oncoproteins, following integration of the viral DNA into the host chromosome. Factors that could increase the risk of the acquisition of oncogenic mutations include smoking and the long-term use of oral contraceptives. Therefore, novel strategies to treat cervical neoplasia are targeting the E6 and E7 proteins, since their overexpression is essential to the maintenance of the oncogenic phenotype (see Chapters 6 and 13).

Further reading

Classon M and Harlow E (2002). The retinoblastoma tumour suppressor in development and cancer. *Nature Reviews Cancer,* **2**: 910–17.

Doorbar J (2006). Molecular biology of human papilloma virus infection and cervical cancer. *Clinical Science*, **110**: 525–41.

Duensing S and Münger K (2004). Mechanisms of genomic instability in human cancer: insights from studies with human papilloma virus oncoproteins. *International Journal of Cancer*, **109**: 157–62.

Goodwin EC and DiMaio D (2000). Repression of human papilloma virus oncogenes in HeLa cervical carcinoma cells causes the orderly reactivation of dormant tumor suppressor pathways. *Proceedings of the National Academy of Science, USA*, **97**: 12513–18.

Howley PM and Lowy DR (2007). Papilloma viruses. In DM Knipe and PM Howley, eds. *Fields virology*. 2nd edition, 2299–354.

Walboomers JM, Jacobs MV, Manos MM, Bosch FX, Kummer JA, et al. (1999). Human papilloma virus is a necessary cause of invasive cervical cancer worldwide. *Journal of Pathology*, **189**: 12–19.

Woodman CBJ, Collins SI, Young LS (2007). The natural history of cervical HPV infection: unresolved issues. *Nature Reviews Cancer*, **7**: 11–22.

Chapter 4

HPV and genital cancer: the essential epidemiology

F Xavier Bosch, Silvia de Sanjosé, and Xavier Castellsagué

Key points

- In spite of screening efforts, cervical cancer remains the second most common cancer in women worldwide. In developed countries, it is the most common cancer in young women.
- HPV DNA is detected on average in 10% of normal cytology and almost in 100% of cervical cancer specimens.
- HPV 16 and 18 account for at least 70% of cancers worldwide. They both induce persistency and progression at a higher rate than other high-risk oncogenic types.
- Human papilloma virus (HPV) transmission occurs largely during sexual intercourse with limited protection from condom use. Other factors influencing progression from HPV infection to advanced high-grade squamous intra-epithelial lesion (HSIL) and cancer include smoking, long-term use of oral contraceptives, high parity, HIV infection, and immunosuppression.
- HPV 16 and other high-risk types are responsible for a sizeable fraction of vulval (20%), vaginal (80%), penile (40%), and anal (90%) cancers. Research is ongoing for cancers of the oropharynx and oral cavity.

4.1 Introduction

The causal role of human papilloma virus (HPV) in all cancers of the uterine cervix has been firmly established biologically (Chapter 3) and epidemiologically. HPV types 16 and 18 account for about 70% of the cases worldwide. HPV has been recognized as a necessary cause of cervical cancer, meaning that in the absence of the persistent presence of HPV DNA in the cervical cells, cervical cancer will not occur. Thus, prevention strategies based on HPV testing in screening programmes (Chapter 1) or HPV type-specific vaccination are based on solid ground (Chapters 7, 8, and 12). Most cancers of the vagina and anus are likewise caused by HPV 16, as are a sizeable fraction of cancers of the penis and of the oropharynx.

4.2 Burden of cancer linked to HPV: The impact of cervical screening

In spite of the opportunities offered by screening programmes, cervical cancer remains the second most common cancer among women worldwide, with an estimated 493 000 new cases and 274 000 deaths in 2002. This is due to the fact that the majority of women in the world do not have access to cervical screening, which can prevent up to 75% of cervical cancer.

Cervical cancer clusters in developing countries where 80% of the cases occur, and it accounts for at least 15% of all female cancers. In some of these populations the cumulative lifetime risk of developing cervical cancer is estimated to be in the range of 1.5–3%, whereas in developed countries it accounts for only 3.6% of all new cancers in women with a cumulative risk of 0.8% up to 65 years of age. In general, the lowest rates (less than 15 per 100 000) are found in Europe (except in many of the Eastern European countries), North America, and Japan. The incidence is particularly high in Latin America (age-standardized incidence rates; ASR 33.5 per 100 000) and the Caribbean (ASR 33.5), sub-Saharan Africa (ASR 31.0), and South-Central (ASR 26.5) and Southeast Asia (ASR 18.3). Moreover, within the developed countries, cervical cancer also clusters in the lower socio-economic strata, signalling the lack of appropriate screening as one of the major determinants of the occurrence of the invasive stages of the disease. Predictions based on the passive growth of the population and the increase in life expectancy indicate that the expected number of cervical cancers in 2020 will increase by 40% worldwide corresponding to 56% in developing countries and 11% in the developed parts of the world.

Mortality rates are substantially lower than incidence. Worldwide, the ratio of mortality to incidence is 55%. The 5-year survival rates vary between regions with good prognosis in developed countries (73% in US registries and 63% in European registries). Because cervical cancer affects relatively young women, it is an important cause of years of life lost (YLL). One recent estimate concluded that cervical cancer is the biggest single cause of YLL from cancer in the developing world. In Latin America, the Caribbean, and Eastern Europe, cervical cancer makes a greater contribution to YLL than diseases such as tuberculosis or acquired immune deficiency syndrome (AIDS). It also makes the largest contribution to YLL from cancer in the populous regions of sub-Saharan Africa and South-Central Asia (see Chapter 10).

4.3 Other cancers linked to HPV infection

Cancers of the vulva and vagina are rare tumors that jointly account for 6–9% of cancers of the genital tract. Although the majority are squamous cell keratinizing carcinomas (>80%), two distinct histological subtypes are recognized. The morphologically warty or basaloid type, which is associated with HPV infection, is diagnosed at relatively younger ages, is often concurrent with precursor lesions of vulval intraepithelial neoplasia (VIN 2/3), and tends to follow the epidemiological pattern of a sexually transmitted origin (related to larger number of partners and a record of previous cervical lesions). In contrast, the keratinizing squamous cell vulvar cancers are diagnosed at older ages, and are often related to chronic degenerative epithelial conditions such as lichen sclerosus.

Cancer of the vagina is consistently rarer than vulval cancer. The majority of cases are preceded by vaginal intraepithelial neoplasia (VAIN 2/3) and HPV; mostly HPV 16 has been implicated in over 90% of the cases.

Cancer of the penis is a rare cancer, accounting for less than 0.5% of cancers in men. The incidence in Jewish populations is particularly low. The importance of circumcision in determining the risk of penile cancer has been evident for many years. Case–control studies estimated that the risk of penile cancer is reduced about threefold among circumcised men. Circumcision also protects against other sexually transmitted infections, such as human immunodeficiency virus (HIV), and recently it has been shown that husband's circumcision also protects women from HPV infections and cervical cancer.

Cancers of the anus are those arising in the anal canal, largely in a zone of transition epithelium similar to the one encountered in the cervix. In most populations, anal cancer is twice as common in females as in males, although the incidence is particularly high amongst homosexual males. HPV 16 is found in 85–95% of the cases and other risk factors include co-infections with HIV, cigarette smoking, frequency of anal intercourse, and the number of lifetime sexual partners.

Current research is actively investigating the role of HPV infections, notably of HPV 16, in cancers of the oropharynx (averaged estimates of 35%) and of the oral cavity (averaged estimates of 20%). The number of cases of HPV-related cancers is shown in Table 4.1.

Table 4.1 HPV attributable cancer worldwide in 2002

Site	Attributable to HPV%	Fraction of HPV 16 and 18 among HPV + cases%	Total number of cancers attributable to HPV	Fraction of all cancer related to HPV%
Cervix	100.00	70.00	492 800	4.54
Penis	40.00	63.00	10500	0.10
Vulva, vagina	40.00	80.00	16 000	0.15
Anus	90.00	92.00	27 300	0.25
Mouth	3.00	95.00	8200	0.08
Oropharynx	12.00	89.00	6200	0.06
			561 100	**5.17**

Source: Parkin DM, et al. 2006

4.4 Burden of HPV infections in women with normal cytology

Two recent sources have provided estimates that may reflect the global HPV prevalence, the age-specific HPV prevalence, and the type specific HPV prevalence as well as an approximation to the international variability. In a centrally coordinated international study, the International Agency for research on Cancer (IARC) provided data from 15 areas in four continents among women aged 15–74. The age-standardized prevalence ranged from a low (less than 5%) in some Mediterranean countries and in some countries in South East Asia to a high (greater than 15%) in several countries in Latin America and in a few populations in Africa.

In a comprehensive review of the literature, with standardized criteria for study inclusion and statistical analyses adjusting for the variables that challenge comparability of studies, the summary estimate of the world's HPV population prevalence among women with normal cytology was 10% with strong geographical variability. The corresponding prevalence in North America was 11%, in Europe 8%, in Asia 8%, in South America 20%, and in Africa 22%.

The age-specific prevalence consistently shows higher proportions among the young age groups, a steep decline in the young adults, and a variable pattern afterwards. In some countries, notably in the Americas, Europe, and Africa, the prevalence increased again in the post-menopausal age groups, whereas in Asia the prevalence remained fairly constant across age groups (Figure 4.1). This pattern strongly reflects the sexual nature of the transmission and the ability of the immune system to cope with the infection in most instances.

Figure 4.1 Age-specific HPV DNA prevalence among women with normal cytology by continent

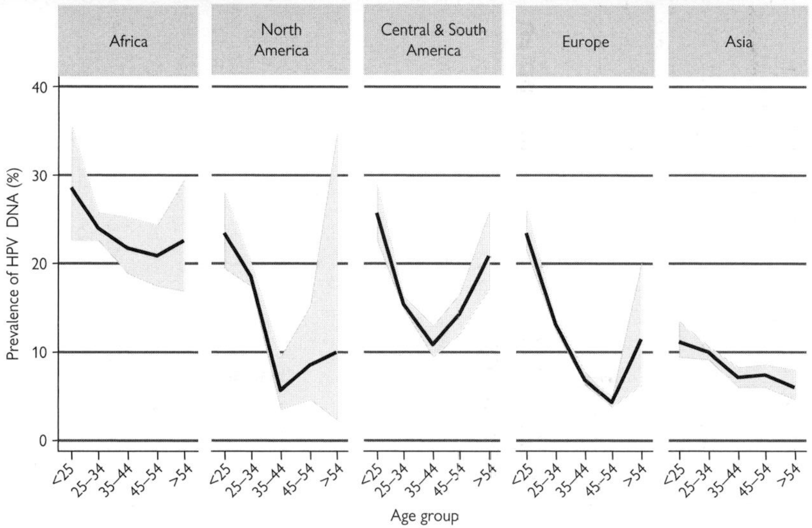

Source: De Sanjosé, et al. *Lancet Infectious Diseases*, 2007.

CHAPTER 4 **HPV and genital cancer**

It is now clear that the true high-risk group for cervical cancer is the fraction of women in whom, for reasons that are unknown, the infections cannot be cleared and remain as persistent carriers of a continuously replicating HPV in the basal membrane of the cervical epithelium (Chapter 6).

4.5 HPV and cancer: Epidemiological connection and assessment of causality

4.5.1 Detection of HPV DNA in cervical cancer tissue: The value of prevalence surveys

Since 1995, it is known that HPV DNA can be identified in virtually all (99.7%) cervical cancer cases and that the fraction of putative HPV negatives in most series of cases is largely due to test limitations or quality of the specimen. Current meta-analyses of the literature show that the most frequent HPV types found in cervical cancer and its relative contribution are fairly stable geographically. Figure 4.2a shows the distribution in the reference IARC's programme and in a recent literature review.

The eight most common HPV types detected in both series, in descending order of frequency, were HPV 16, 18, 45, 31, 33, 52, 58, and 35, and these are responsible for about 90% of all cervical cancers worldwide. The distribution is very similar to the pre-invasive lesions (high-grade squamous intraepithelial lesion, HSIL). The distribution of HPV types for adenocarcinoma (ADC) is slightly different in that HPV 18 plays a more important role (up to 30% of the types) and globally HPV 16, 18, and 45 account for over 85% of the ADC cases. This is of interest, since ADC tends to escape early detection in cytology-based screening programmes, and HPV 16 and 18 vaccines could offer wider protection. Figure 4.2b shows the relative contribution of each HPV type to the burden of cervical cancer worldwide.

4.5.2 Comparing the prevalence of HPV DNA in cervical cancer cases and a control group: The contribution of case–control studies

Case–control studies have contributed powerful methodology in cancer epidemiology to estimate the risk of disease (cervical cancer), given the relevant exposure (HPV). Risk estimates are expressed as Odds Ratio (OR) [and as relative risk (RR) in prospective cohort studies], both of which express the factor (the magnitude of the OR or the RR) by which any given women multiply their risk (probability) of cervical cancer if exposed to the relevant cause (HPV). *The principle of case–control studies is that the probability of disease–given exposure is equivalent to the probability of exposure–given disease.* The former

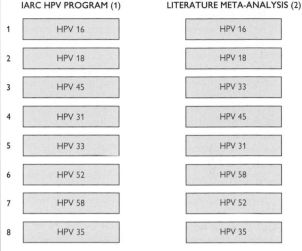

Figure 4.2a **The eight most common HPV types in cervical cancer—worldwide estimates**

IARC HPV PROGRAM (1)	LITERATURE META-ANALYSIS (2)
1	HPV 16	HPV 16
2	HPV 18	HPV 18
3	HPV 45	HPV 33
4	HPV 31	HPV 45
5	HPV 33	HPV 31
6	HPV 52	HPV 58
7	HPV 58	HPV 52
8	HPV 35	HPV 35

Sources: Muñoz N, Bosch FX, *et al. International Journal of Cancer*, 2004; and Smith J, *et al. Journal of Virology*, 2007.

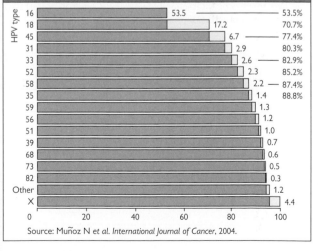

Figure 4.2b **The global contribution of each HPV type to the burden of cervical cancer. Weighed estimate by study size and cervical cancer incidence**

HPV type	value	cumulative
16	53.5	53.5%
18	17.2	70.7%
45	6.7	77.4%
31	2.9	80.3%
33	2.6	82.9%
52	2.3	85.2%
58	2.2	87.4%
35	1.4	88.8%
59	1.3	
56	1.2	
51	1.0	
39	0.7	
68	0.6	
73	0.5	
82	0.3	
Other	1.2	
X	4.4	

Source: Muñoz N *et al. International Journal of Cancer*, 2004.

(to estimate the probability of disease–given exposure) requires follow-up of exposed and unexposed persons; the latter (to estimate the probability of exposure–given disease) allows retrospective assessment of exposure in cases that are currently occurring (provided validated methods of assessing exposure, for example by examining the presence of HPV DNA in cervical cells, exist) and its comparison to the presence of the same exposure in a group of individuals serving as controls. These controls are traditionally sampled from a universe of healthy individuals of similar key characteristics such as age, sex, and place of residency. Some technical qualifiers of these definitions and methods of statistical analyses are of importance, and excellent references are available. Figure 4.3 summarizes the prevalence of HPV DNA among cases and controls and the corresponding adjusted ORs for squamous cell carcinomas (SCC) and for ADC/adenosquamous cell carcinomas of the cervix.

Figure 4.4 shows the type-specific risk estimates for the five most common HPV types in cervical cancer. As shown by the overlapping of the confidence intervals, the risk linked to any of the rest of the high-risk types is statistically equal to the very high risk linked to HPV 16 or 18. The observation extends to the other 15 types that are detected as single infections in cervical cancer and formed the theoretical background for introducing cocktail testing in screening programmes. The clinical assumption is that management of a woman found HPV high-risk positive would be identical irrespective of the specific type. Notably, the risk of women in whom multiple types are identified (i.e. 16 & 18) does not differ from the risk of women with single infections. The observation reinforces the concept that there is no interaction between HPV types in accelerating (or modulating) progression to advanced cancer.

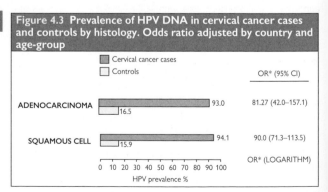

Figure 4.3 Prevalence of HPV DNA in cervical cancer cases and controls by histology. Odds ratio adjusted by country and age-group

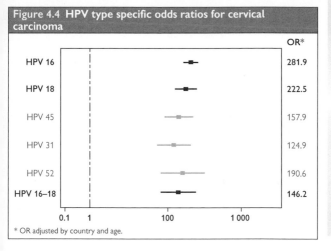

Figure 4.4 HPV type specific odds ratios for cervical carcinoma

	OR*
HPV 16	281.9
HPV 18	222.5
HPV 45	157.9
HPV 31	124.9
HPV 52	190.6
HPV 16–18	146.2

0.1   1   100   1 000

* OR adjusted by country and age.

4.5.3 Observing the development of (pre-invasive) cases in women exposed to HPV

Cohort studies allow prospective observations of pre-cancer development and compare absolute risk of progression (proportion of women developing a new high-grade cytological abnormality within the interval) among women with normal cytology at study entry with and without exposure to HPV (HPV DNA positive in exfoliated cervical cells). The risk is expressed as RR and is interpreted in the same way as ORs are interpreted. Cohort prospective studies require longer periods of observation due to the long incubation period between exposure to HPV and the development of cytological abnormality and repeated visits with sampling because of the asymptomatic nature of the intermediate end points. From natural history studies the currently accepted relevant end points are the persistence of HPV (at least two tests positives at 6- to 12+ month interval), low-grade squamous intraepithelial lesion (LSIL) and most importantly, high-grade squamous intraepithelial lesion (HSIL), the only end point accepted so far by the World Health Organisation (WHO) and some of the regulatory agencies to assess HPV vaccine efficacy. Ethical considerations preclude the completion of studies that continue clinical observation until the stage of invasive cancer.

Figure 4.5 shows that women who are normal in their cytology but positive for HPV DNA (16 or 18) at study entry, have a higher absolute probability (close to 20%) of evolving to CIN 3+ in a 10-year time interval than do women exposed to other high-risk types (around 5%) and much higher than do unexposed women (less than 1%).

44

Figure 4.5 Cumulative incidence of CIN 3+ in a follow-up study of 13 000 women over a 10-year period by a single HPV test result at enrolment

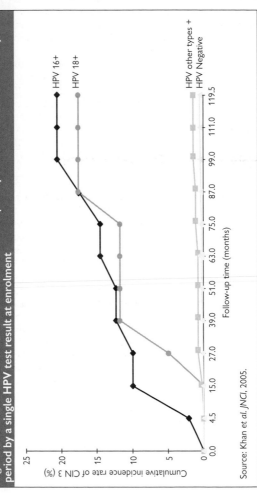

HPV 16+

HPV 18+

HPV other types +

HPV Negative

Follow-up time (months)

Cumulative incidence rate of CIN 3 (%)

Source: Khan et al. JNCI, 2005.

Further, similar studies that tested repeatedly for HPV in the follow-up interval clearly indicated that persistent infection is a significant factor in the progression probability. In Denmark, women who tested HPV positive for a high-risk type twice in a 10-year interval progressed to CIN 3+ at 800-fold the progression rate observed in an equivalent group of HPV-negative women. Women who tested HPV positive transiently showed an intermediate risk of progression, signalling that in situations in which HPV DNA cannot be consistently detected evidence of some level of exposure to HPV could still reflect the risk of developing CIN 3+. In some of these studies, CIN 2/3 developed within 2 years of first HPV DNA detection, thus indicating that, contrary to the theory that prolonged periods of HPV infection are necessary for progression to CIN 2/3, these precancerous lesions can develop, albeit rarely, as an early manifestation of HPV infection, at least in young women.

4.6 **Risk factors for HPV infection**

The risk of cervical cancer has been historically linked to the number of sexual partners, early age at sexual initiation, and to the number of partners of the husband or male partner. Male homosexuals are at high risk of anal infections and anal cancer. These observations clearly indicated that genital HPV infections are sexually transmitted, although intercourse with full penetration is not a requisite. HPV viruses circulate with and within the exfoliated cells from the infected epithelia and are often a field infection, including the genital and perineal skin. Thus condoms, particularly if used irregularly, only offer partial protection. Anecdotal reports of transmission by fingers or fomites are available.

HPV infections occur with a high-attack rate soon after sexual initiation. Follow-up studies of virgins from different countries after sexual debut have shown up to 70% of women becoming HPV DNA positive at least once within 48 months. The cumulative lifetime exposure to HPV has been estimated to be close to 80% and for HPV 16 or 18 it is 20%. Thus, primary prevention with HPV vaccines should focus on the years before sexual initiation, in the adolescent and pre-adolescent age groups.

Mother-to-child transmission has been reported in a limited manner. Less than 5% of HPV-infected mothers transmit the infection to the oral cavity or the external genital of the newborns, but these infections are usually transient and no clinical outcomes have been reported. One exception is the transmission of HPV 6 and 11 from infected mothers to the newborn. HPV 6 and 11 are responsible for 90% of the genital warts (GW), and when transmission to the respiratory tract of the newborn occurs during birth the infection can evolve into recurrent respiratory papillomatosis (RRP), a condition that requires frequent surgical interventions to clear the airways. Papillomas can eventually expand to the rest of the respiratory tract and occasionally (1–3%) cause severe complications and death.

4.7 Risk factors for progression from HPV persistent infection to cancer

Although many women are exposed to cervical HPV infections, most do not progress to cervical cancer. The potential cofactors could be classed as environmental or exogenous and host factors. The environmental factors include hormones, tobacco smoking, and co-infection with other sexually transmitted agents; viral characteristics, such as HPV type or HPV variants, viral load at the time of the infection, and viral integration are often included. Host cofactors include endogenous hormones, genetic factors, and other factors related to the immune response. There is growing evidence that the initial immune response to the infection is the key determinant of the prognosis in its initial stages. Environmental factors have been identified as capable of modulating progression from infection to neoplasia and invasion. The evaluation of these progression factors are based on the comparison of cases and controls, including only the controls that are also HPV positive but without disease (HPV-restricted case–control studies).

Hormonal contraceptives: The IARC monograph on hormones and cancer classed combined oral contraceptives as carcinogenic to the cervix. The risk of invasive cervical cancer increases with increasing duration of oral contraceptive use but declines with time since stopping so that by 10 or more years after stopping use, the risk has returned to that of never users. The hypothesized mechanism through which hormonal contraceptives may act as a cofactor is through the effect of oestrogens or progestogens, enhancing HPV gene-expression in the cervix via progesterone-receptor mechanisms and hormone-response elements in the viral genome.

High parity: Consistent with the results showing an implication of hormonal factors in the HPV-related carcinogenesis of the cervix, the number of full-term pregnancies has been associated with an increased risk of invasive cervical carcinoma after adjustment for number of sexual partners and age at first intercourse. The RR for invasive cervical cancer increases by 10% with each additional full-term pregnancy and with each year of decreasing age at first full-term pregnancy.

Tobacco smoking: The monograph programme at IARC has classified tobacco smoking as a cause of cervical cancer, and virtually all case–control studies on smoking and cervical cancer have reported increased risk among smokers. The association is less clear with

ADC of the cervix which shares some epidemiological traits with the endometrial ADC.

Other sexually transmitted agents as cofactors in cervical carcinogenesis: The specific role of other infectious agents in the pathogenesis of cervical cancer has been studied in many epidemiological studies. The most studied sexually transmitted infectious agents for which some evidence has been shown in relation to cervical cancer are herpes simplex virus-2 (HSV-2), Chlamydia Trachomatis (CT), and HIV. Of these, HIV infections and AIDS-related immunosuppression is the single co-infection that consistently shown to increase the likelihood of being HPV positive and to progress to cervical cancer. This association appears to be stronger for women with a low CD4 T-lymphocyte count. Women infected with both HIV and HPV are at a higher risk of squamous intraepithelial lesions (SILs) than women infected with either of the two viruses separately. HIV-infected men and women show higher incidence rates of anal HPV infection, anal intraepithelial neoplasia (AIN), and anal cancer. The central role of immune response has also been assessed in cases of medically induced immunosuppression among organ transplant recipients, a critical group at increased risk of HPV-associated anogenital cancers compared with age-matched healthy individuals.

4.8 Conclusion

The global burden of cervical cancer remains high in the world, notably in developing countries without screening programmes. The aetiology of the disease has been linked to persistent infections with a limited number of HPV types. Novel options for protection take advantage of the technology for HPV DNA identification and of the ability to use highly efficient vaccines against the most relevant of the HPV types.

Further reading

Bosch FX, Cuzick J, Schiller J, *et al.* (2006). HPV vaccines and screening in the prevention of cervical cancer. *Vaccine*, **24**(suppl. 3) (available also in Spanish): S1–S264.

Castellsagué X, Diaz M, de Sanjose S, *et al.* (2006). Worldwide human papilloma virus etiology of cervical adenocarcinoma and its cofactors: implications for screening and prevention. *Journal of National Cancer Institute*, **98**: 303–15.

de Sanjosé S, Diaz M, Castellsague X, *et al.* (2007). Worldwide prevalence and genotype distribution of cervical human papilloma virus DNA in women with normal cytology: a meta-analysis. *Lancet Infectious Diseases*, **7**: 453–9.

Dos Santos Silva I (1999). *Cancer epidemiology: principles and methods.* International Agency for Research on Cancer, Lyon.

Parkin DM (2006). The global health burden of infection-associated cancers in the year 2000. *International Journal of Cancer*, **118**: 3030–44.

Smith JS, Lindsay L, Hoots B, *et al.* (2007). Human papilloma virus type distribution in invasive cervical cancer and high-grade cervical lesions: a meta-analysis update. *International Journal of Cancer*, **121**: 621–32.

Walboomers JM, Jacobs MV, Manos MM, *et al.* (1999). Human papilloma virus is a necessary cause of invasive cervical cancer worldwide. *Journal of Pathology*, **189**: 12–9.

Chapter 5

The role of HPV testing in cervical screening

Margaret E Cruickshank

Key points

- The knowledge that high-risk human papilloma virus (HPV) infection is necessary to develop cervical cancer has prompted the exploration of its utility in cervical screening.
- HPV testing could be for triage of low-grade smears to improve the sensitivity of cytology alone, and select women at most risk who require colposcopy.
- The sensitivity and specificity of HPV testing relate to the threshold of the test, and the underlying prevalence of cervical intraepithelial neoplasia (CIN) in the tested population.
- The role of HPV testing in primary screening holds promise because of high sensitivity, but its lack of specificity will need to be addressed before it could be recommended to replace cytology as an initial screen.
- HPV testing has been shown to detect residual disease following treatment of CIN earlier than cytology. Its use as a test of cure will allow earlier return to routine recall for most women.

5.1 Rationale for testing

Cervical screening in organized population-based programmes has been successful in reducing the incidence of cervical cancer. As we strive to reduce this further, our ambition has to be balanced against any risks that result from screening, such as referral to colposcopy, treatment, and resultant anxiety. The limitations of cervical cytology, particularly in terms of sensitivity, are well known. If we were only to investigate women with high-grade smears, we could reduce the number of false-positive results (see Table 5.1), but at the cost of missing some women with disease. We can increase the sensitivity of the test by investigating women with low-grade changes (borderline nuclear abnormalities and mild dyskaryosis in the United Kingdom), but this inevitably increases the number of women with a false-positive result as the incidence of cervical intraepithelial neoplasia (CIN) will be lower in this group. Many women with low-grade abnormalities may undergo investigation to determine the presence or absence of CIN; the colposcopy services have to cope with increased workload, with no impact on cervical cancer.

Considerable work has been done to optimize cytological screening, including quality assurance, bench marking, and the introduction of liquid-based cytology (LBC). The characterization of morphological changes in cervical cells, however, remains subjective with marked intra- and inter-observer variability in reporting. A molecular test for HPV DNA avoids these limitations with a quantitative result based on a predetermined cut-off and with good reproducibility of the test results.

High-risk human papilloma virus (HR HPV) is necessary for most high-grade CIN lesions and all cervical cancers (Chapters 3 and 4). In addition to the importance of high-risk genotypes which are more common in high-grade CIN and cancer (e.g. 16, 18, 31, 33, 45, and 52), these types are also more likely to persist in the cervix than lower-risk types. The long natural history of cervical cancer starts with HPV

Table 5.1 Understanding test performance[*]	
Sensitivity	Tells us how good a test is at detecting those individuals who have disease by providing the proportion of those with disease who test positive
Specificity	Tells us how good a test is at detecting those individuals who do not have disease by providing the proportion of those who are disease free and test negative
Positive predictive value (PPV)	Tells us what proportion of women who test positive actually have disease
Negative predictive value (NPV)	Tells us what proportion of women who test negative are actually disease free

[*] The ideal screening test would be virtually 100% sensitive and 100% specific with positive and negative predictive values close to 100%. In practice this is impossible to achieve; sensitivity and positive predictive value close to 100% usually necessitates a lower specificity and negative predictive value, and vice versa.

infection, HPV persistence, and the development of pre-invasive disease (CIN). HPV testing will therefore not only identify virtually all women with high grade CIN, it will also detect those with persistent or transient infection. Although the latter two groups are at increased risk over time, HPV screening could generate a group of the 'worried-well', creating unnecessary anxiety.

5.2 Triage of low-grade smear

Only 20% of low-grade cytology contains HR HPV, but low-risk HPV types are often identified. Earlier cross-sectional studies have shown that those women with a low-grade smear but underlying high CIN could be identified by HPV testing. The utility of HPV testing in detecting disease is higher for lower grades of abnormality. A positive result could be used to triage women either to colposcopy if HPV positive, or back to cervical surveillance if HPV negative, with the expectation that their smears will regress to normal as they are not at risk of developing disease. This avoids delays in the investigation and management of women who are most likely to have or develop high-grade CIN whilst avoiding further interventions to confirm normality for women without significant disease. Many European, Scandinavian, and North American countries have conducted clinical trials on HPV triage. The largest, Ascus/LSIL Triage Study (ALTS), found that women with low-grade squamous intraepithelial lesion (LSIL) (approximates to mild dyskaryosis) are usually HPV positive and was judged to have no additional benefit in HPV testing. However, women with atypical squamous cells of undetermined significance (ASCUS) (approximates to borderline) could be reflex tested for HPV and only referred to colposcopy if they are HPV positive.

Longer-term follow-up in other triage studies had not identified superiority between reflex testing and cytology alone, but HPV testing allows earlier diagnosis of high-grade CIN. This is advantageous if the interval to the next screening round and the number of women who can be returned to routine recall are increased. In addition, this provides reassurance to the women without the necessity for clinical interventions.

HPV testing may be less useful in women under the age of 30 for triage because of the high prevalence of HR HPV in younger women, however, CIN is most prevalent between 25 and 30 years. This triage will result in an increased number of colposcopies, with only 15–25% having CIN2 or worse. HPV infection, even when associated with CIN, may merely indicate a very early lesion that may not be identified by colposcopy and biopsy. If the women were not at any increased risk of progression within the time scale of the next screening round, early detection would not directly benefit them. HPV triage could, therefore, be optimized by restricting its use to selected high-risk groups such as women over the age of 30 or with persistence of HR HPV genotypes. On the other hand, having a different management for women of different ages adds complexity to a screening programme. Furthermore, HPV triage at 25 years would accelerate the diagnosis of prevalent high-grade CIN for women who are entering screening.

There is a financial cost to a policy of HPV triage because all women require two tests, smear and HPV. This would be offset by reducing the number of women who require colposcopy and repeat cytology as a result of the protection associated with being HPV negative. HPV typing using a restricted set of high-risk types could select a smaller proportion for colposcopy, but this would reduce sensitivity.

5.3 **Primary screening**

Since HPV is a sensitive but non-specific test for high grade CIN, it could be useful in first-line screening but many women who test positive would not have disease.

Two large randomized trials of HPV testing in primary screening have recently been reported from the Netherlands and Sweden and the results of others are awaited. Both trials compared conventional cytology alone with conventional cytology plus HPV testing over two screening rounds. Both showed similar results in that the co-testing detected more high-grade CIN in the initial (prevalence) round but there was no difference between arms over the two rounds combined. These results need to be confirmed with liquid based cytology. HPV testing therefore, does achieve greater sensitivity with respect to conventional cytology but the means of managing women who are cytology negative/HPV positive would need to be resolved. Furthermore, given that cervical screening takes place over repeated rounds, the failure to increase detection rates over two rounds combined, certainly casts doubt on the cost effectiveness of co-testing. HPV testing triaged by cytology could be cost effective if other savings can be made; for example, through lengthened screening intervals.

5.4 **Test of cure following treatment of CIN**

The use of HPV testing in the follow-up of women after the local treatment of CIN is strongly supported by clinical evidence. Follow-up is essential post-treatment both to ensure the success of treatment and to detect any recurrence of new disease. Women remain at increased risk of recurrent CIN for at least 8 years but possibly much longer. Over 90% of women are successfully treated but all are asked to comply with prolonged follow-up to confirm cure. In reality, some women default from 10 years of annual smears and so remain at risk. Initial evidence indicated that local treatment often eradicated HPV infection and recognized that some women remained HPV positive. Both retrospective and prospective studies confirm that HPV testing can identify around 15% of women who remain HR HPV positive and who need to remain on surveillance. HPV detection may indicate residual microscopic foci of disease that cytology and colposcopy are too insensitive to detect. Persistence of HR HPV in a transformation zone (TZ) susceptible to atypia can progress to recurrent disease. As there are currently no therapeutic options to eradicate HPV, we must continue to rely on available tools for follow-up—cytology and colposcopy. If recurrence is not identified, further surveillance may require repeat HPV testing to identify persistence and ongoing risk. Crucially, the large majority of women who are HPV negative after treatment are at such low risk of residual or developing new disease within 3 years, that they can probably be safely returned to routine recall. This provides much earlier reassurance both for the woman and the clinician than is currently available.

5.5 **Screening prior to vaccination**

Much of the current data on the protection given by HPV vaccination relates to the women who have been pretested in clinical trials to exclude current HPV infection with the vaccine types. There are concerns regarding the benefit of vaccinating women who have already been exposed to HPV. The short-term data available have indicated the benefit of protection from the other HPV vaccine types and some cross-protection against non-vaccine HPV types which are closely related to HPV 16 and 18, HPV 31 and 45 (Chapters 6–8). We know that HPV infections are common and women can be re-infected with the same HPV types. The point prevalence of HPV 16 and 18 co-existing for an individual woman, however, is low, in the region of only 1–2%. It does not make clinical or economic sense to pre-screen all women by HPV testing for 16/18 when over 90% would be protected for 16/18 associated CIN.

Further reading

Arbyn M, Paraskevaidis E, Martin-Hirsch P, Prendiville W, Dillner J (2005). Clinical utility of HPV-DNA detection: triage of minor cervical lesions, follow-up of women treated for high-grade CIN: an update of pooled evidence. *Gynecologic Oncology*, **99**(3 Suppl 1): S7–11.

Bulkeman's NWJ, Berkhof J, Rozendaal L, Van Kemenande FJ, Boeke AJP, Bulk S, Verheijn RHM, Van Gronigen K, Boon ME, Ruitinga W, Van Ballegooijen M, Snijders PJF, Meijer CJLM (2007). Human Papilloma virus DNA testing for the detection of cervical intraepithelial neoplasia grade 3:5 year follow-up of a randomized, controlled, implementation trial. *Lancet*, **370**: 1764–72.

Davies P, Arbyn M, Dillner J, *et al.* (2006). A report on the current status of European research on the use of human papilloma virus testing for primary cervical cancer screening. *International Journal of Cancer*, **118**: 791–6.

Kitchener HC, Almonte M, Wheeler P, *et al.* (ARTISTIC Trial Study Group) (2006). HPV testing in routine cervical screening: cross sectional data from the ARTISTIC trial. *British Journal of Cancer*, **95**: 56–61.

Naucler P, Ryd W, Tönberg S, Strand A, Wadell G, Elfgren K, Rådberg T, Strander B, Forstlund O, Hansson B-G, Rylander E, and Dillner J. (2007). Human Papilloma Virus and Papanicolaou Tests to screen for Cervical Cancer. *New England Journal of Medicine*, **357**: 1589–97.

Paraskevaidis E, Arbyn M, Sotiriadis A, *et al.* (2004). The role of HPV DNA testing in the follow-up period after treatment for CIN: a systematic review of the literature. *Cancer Treatment Reviews*, **30**: 205–11.

Ronco G, Cuzick J, Segnan N, *et al.* (NTCC working group). (2007). HPV triage for low grade (L-SIL) cytology is appropriate for women over 35 in mass cervical cancer screening using liquid based cytology. *European Journal of Cancer*, **43**: 476–80.

Part 3

Immune control of HPV infection in cervical neoplasia

Chapter 6

Natural immune control of HPV infection

Peter L Stern

Key points

- Most human papilloma virus (HPV) infections in the cervix are naturally controlled. Initially this utilizes the innate immune response.
- Innate immunity is mediated by cytokines such as interferon, produced by epithelial cells and antigen-presenting cells (APCs) or by lytic cells such as natural killer cells and macrophages which also produce cytokines.
- APCs (e.g. dendritic cells) sense the local environment and transfer information about the HPV infection to the local lymph node to activate the adaptive immune response.
- Optimally, a balance of T helper cell 1 and 2 types of response facilitates the development of both HPV-specific cytotoxic T cells (CTLs) and support for production of virus neutralizing antibodies by B cells.
- Adaptive immunity provides the specificity of the immune weapons, their expansion, and provision of immunological memory.
- Long-term control depends on memory B and T cells to provide a rapid delivery of cell-mediated immunity or neutralizing antibodies to halt any new virus infection at an early stage.

6.1 The battleground—the virus strategy of attack

A human papilloma virus (HPV) infection exploits the life cycle of the differentiating epithelium of its target tissue; in the cervix this is the transformation zone (TZ). The infectious cycle of HPV involves reprogramming the cell to permit virus replication and viral particle production. Although the cytological changes associated with infection or CIN are well characterized and exploited in the screening programme, the precise reactions of the host's immune response have been much harder to ascertain, principally because the important events occur locally and with unknown timing. This is further complicated by the manner in which the immune response evolves to combat the different stages of disease which may occur over weeks/months (infection), months/years (CIN), or years/decades (cancer) (Figure 6.1).

The virus utilizes specific viral genes and the machinery of the host's differentiating cells from stem to squamous cells to complete its life cycle, and it manages this without any significant disruption to the tissue. Thus the sentinel cells (antigen presenting cells (APCs) called dendritic cells) and other innate immune cells that can detect elements of tissue damage or pathogens using Toll-like-receptors (TLRs) can fail to notice infection. Activation of the innate immunity is the means to activate the adaptive immune system, so without the appropriate signals via the sentinel cells, the adaptive immune system remains on stand by. Importantly, if the APCs sample HPV infection but are not properly activated they can send negative signals to the adaptive immune mechanisms, which could otherwise combat the infection.

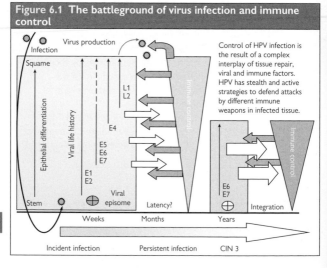

Figure 6.1 **The battleground of virus infection and immune control**

Control of HPV infection is the result of a complex interplay of tissue repair, viral and immune factors. HPV has stealth and active strategies to defend attacks by different immune weapons in infected tissue.

This stealth strategy allows HPV to remain under the radar of the host and facilitates the establishment of a productive infection. In addition, the viral E6 and E7 genes modulate the infected cells' sensitivity to anti-viral responses of the tissue such as production of interferons. If infection persists, the viral genome can become integrated into the cellular genes and this can lead to a failure to respond to apoptotic signals (programmed cell death) and thus immortality. This situation is characterized by increased expression of viral E6 and E7 oncoproteins that interfere with cell processes, which guard the host genome by delaying DNA replication if genes are damaged, thereby allowing adequate time for their repair. Thus when errors occur, any variant cells can, if advantaged in some way, including avoiding the immune system or ability to spread, etc., develop into a cervical cancer. Fortunately, this is a rather rare and late complication of a persistent HPV infection.

That the immune system has an important part to play in controlling HPV infection is apparent from observations showing that individuals with iatrogenic immunosuppression or primary immunodeficiencies are predisposed to squamous carcinoma and HPV infection. Furthermore, antibodies to animal papilloma viruses have been shown to protect against infection with the virus, and HPV oncogene products have been used as targets for inducing tumour immunity in animal models.

6.2 The battle ground—the immune defence

Immune control of an infection is a derivative from the complex interplay of the innate (non-specific) and the adaptive mechanisms delivered by specific antibodies and cellular effectors (e.g. T cells). The key features of the adaptive immune response are the ability to recognize a pathogen specifically, amplify this activity, and retain the memory so that if the pathogen is encountered again it can be dealt with more efficiently. The latter processes clearly take time, and the innate responses are there to fight any pathogen as the first line of defence. Importantly, the adaptive immune system is activated only if it gets the correct signals from the innate immune system (Figure 6.2).

6.2.1 Innate immunity

The innate immune system includes monocytes, macrophages, polymorphic leucocytes, natural killer cells, and the sentinel dendritic cells. These cells can sense the presence of molecules usually sequestered inside cells and/or derived from pathogens such as high mannose structures, heat shock proteins, DNA, RNA, etc., following infection/tissue damage using a variety of TLRs. This sensing of danger is an important regulator of immune control since on the one hand it

Figure 6.2 Innate and adaptive immune control: the players

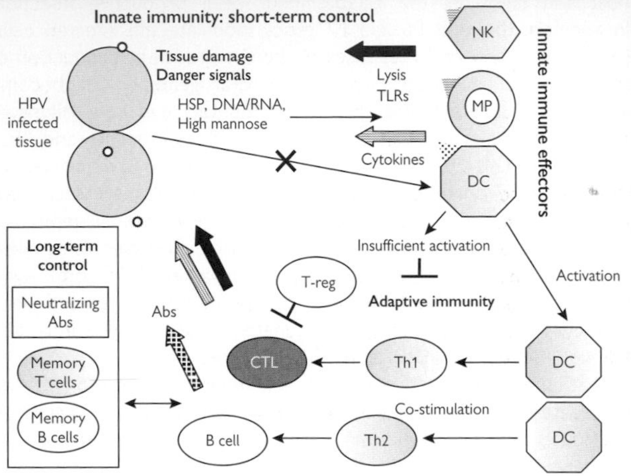

NK = Natural killer cell; MP = Macrophage; DC = Dendritic cell; TLRs= Toll-like-receptors; HSP = Heat Shock Protein; T-reg = T regulatory cell; Th1 or 2 = T cell helper type 1 or 2 response; CTL = cytotoxic T cell; Abs = antibodies.

allows the body to react quickly to real threats but on the other ignores other micro-organisms which do not warrant an immune reaction. HPV, with its life cycle associated with normal desquamation processes, does not cause death of the host cell and has no viraemia, and the infectious virus particles are shed from mucosal surfaces. The process of initial infection is believed to occur following microtrauma of the transformation zone (TZ) of the cervix, with the virus particles interacting with basal cells that sit on a basement membrane. Overall, the stealth strategy of the virus is to avoid providing, at least initially, the important signals associated with inflammation of damaged tissue that activate the innate immune response. When innate immune effectors are activated they provide both cytokine (e.g. interferons) and/or direct cell lysis of the infected cells. It is possible that innate immunity can clear an HPV infection in some cases but it is very likely that in others, HPV genomes in basal cells can provide a continued reservoir of the infection. It is the activation of adaptive immunity which recruits reinforcements to the battlefield and new weaponry with which to neutralize the virus particles and eliminate the infected cells using specific killer T cells. The innate immunity dendritic cells sense the local environment and transfer information about the HPV infection to the local lymph nodes to activate the adaptive immune response.

6.2.2 **Adaptive immunity**

Adaptive HPV-specific cellular immunity is judged critical in the clearance of established infection, since evidence of HPV infection can be presented by HLA molecules (tissue type) on the surface of infected cells. The T cell receptors recognize a complex of virally derived peptides and HLA molecules. Dendritic cells have efficient antigen processing mechanisms which generate the viral peptide–HLA complexes which can be presented in conjunction with particular co-stimulatory molecules to activate the appropriate HPV specific T cells in the lymph nodes. Optimally, this process provides for a balance of T helper 1 and 2 type responses (mediated by different cytokines) leading to the appropriate activation of HPV-specific cytotoxic T cells (CTLs) and support for production of virus neutralizing antibodies by B cells. In this process, the effector T cells receive direction to the infected site where they can deliver a therapeutic payload. The life history of the virus only produces viral particles in the terminally differentiated and dead cells so the target cells of the virus infection which are probably stem cells in the basal layer, can retain the viral genome as a latent infection. The latter is where the viral genome(s) are present in a cell, although essentially undetectable and in a dormant state. To fully clear any infection, virus-specific killer T cells are required, because they can recognize the intracellular viral early gene products which are displayed as HLA-peptide complexes at the cell surface and destroy them directly by cytotoxic mechanisms or indirectly through release of interferons or other cytokines. The virus has already initiated strategies to reduce sensitivity of the infected cell to interferons and it can also reduce the HLA expression, making it harder for any virus-specific T cells to recognize the targets. There is evidence that repertoires of T cells in women with persistent HPV infections and high-grade CIN are depleted of activity against the HPV proteins E2 and E6, whereas E6 specific T cells are detectable in women whose lesions have regressed. These conclusions are mainly the result of analysing the immune cells of the peripheral blood, and this may not always reflect the local conditions most relevant to the control of the HPV-associated lesions. A successful cellular immune reaction will also generate memory T cells to deal with any subsequent infection.

Antibodies are produced by B cells with the target antigens recognized in the manner of a lock-and-key fit. In an HPV infection only the viral particles are extracellular so useful antibodies are ones that can neutralize the viruses. Memory B cells provide the ability to immediately produce more such specific antibodies on subsequent infection but local levels of such molecules could be very important in preventing any infection. How such protection is delivered at the mucosal surface is believed to be through mechanisms that transudate antibodies to the cervical mucus or by serous exudation following local trauma, which provides the route of entry for viral particles to initiate an infection. In either case, effective serological immunity will critically depend on the levels of antibodies found in the plasma. Thus antibody-mediated humoral immunity acts to clear free virus particles and may help protect against re-infection with the same type of HPV; but the antibodies that neutralize are type specific so they offer reduced or no protection against other strains of the virus. It seems likely that at least some women who fail to develop antibodies against HPV after infection must have cleared their infection using only innate mechanisms. Indeed this might be the case even where one subsequently sees the generation of adaptive immunity involving neutralizing antibodies of IgG type against the virus particles and/or T cells recognizing early proteins of the virus genome, including the oncogenes E6 and E7. The lag time between infection with HPV and production of antibodies reinforces the part that innate immunity plays initially and also the effectiveness of viral immune evasion tactics (Table 6.1).

Table 6.1 The immune armoury	
• Danger signals	• Tissue damages sensed through Toll-like receptors (TLRs)
• Innate immune effectors	• Keratinocytes, APC (DC), MP, and NK cells release interferons/ cytokines and/or are cytotoxic (lytic) for infected cells
• Activation of adaptive immune response	• DCs when activated go to local lymph node and depending on balance of signals received in infection activate different types of HPV-specific T cells
• Adaptive immune effectors and regulators	• DC influence balance of effector function generated, including killer T cells (CTLs), neutralizing antibodies or T regulatory cells which can limit useful immunity. If DCs are not activated properly they can anergize any HPV-sepcific response
• Long-term control	• Depends on HPV-specific T and B memory cells to rapidly generate antibodies to neutralize virus particles or to eliminate virus-infected cells.

6.3 **Persistence of HPV infection: A viral attack and immune defence stalemate**

In some individuals the innate immune response is not properly activated and the dendritic cells take signals to their waiting T cell armies in the lymph node, telling them to mothball their weapons (HPV-specific T cells are anergized). In the face of persistent infection, CIN, and ultimately an invasive cancer, the oncogenes E6 and E7 are constitutively expressed and chronic stimulation of the effectors without appropriate immune co-stimulation can also lead to anergy. Another consequence of chronic stimulation can be the generation of T regulatory cells, which are part of the natural control systems built into immune responses to limit and reduce the levels of virus-specific cellular immunity when the danger has passed. These effectors can suppress the activity of CTLs either directly or by the production of cytokines such as IL10 and TGF beta. Emerging evidence has shown increased numbers of these cells in tumours of different types, including those of the cervix. Finally, high-grade lesions and tumour cells can lose the expression of HLA molecules and such cells will have an advantage as the T cell effectors specific for the oncogenes will be impotent since the target will have no cell surface HLA–HPV peptide complexes for the T cell receptor (TCR) to recognize. In some circumstances, the balance of positive and negative immune factors may be changed so that the lesions can be cleared. This is an area where therapeutic vaccines against HPV targets may be of value (see Chapter 13). Figure 6.3 summarizes how the balance of immune system responses versus viral immune evasion mechanisms affects HPV persistence and hence likelihood of disease progression or regression. There remain many questions about the precise details and kinetics of the various immune processes across the natural history of cervical neoplasia and in particular the reasons why immune control fails in some individuals, increasing the likelihood of progression. Some of these are listed in Box 6.1.

6.4 **The realities of immune control**

Clearly HPV infection in young women is very frequent and high-risk HPV 16 and 18 infections, if they persist, carry the principal risk for developing cervical neoplasia, but mostly these are cleared naturally. Emerging data suggest that many women in fact show evidence of second and subsequent infections of, for example, HPV 16. It is important to understand that any documentation of HPV-negative or -positive cytology from the cervix is a hostage to the methodology and its sensitivity which in turn is limited by the frequency of sampling

Figure 6.3 **The balance of virus infection, immune control, and cervical neoplasia**

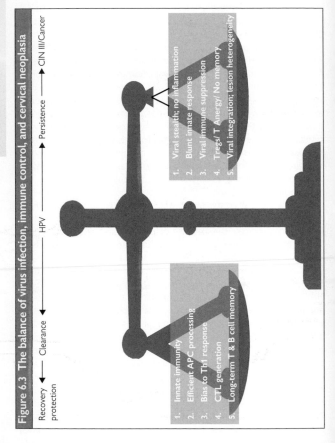

Recovery ◀── Clearance ──── HPV ──── Persistence ──── ▶ CIN III/Cancer
protection

1. Innate immunity
2. Efficient APC processing
3. Bias to Th1 response
4. CTL generation
5. Long-term T & B cell memory

1. Viral stealth; no inflammation
2. Blunt innate response
3. Viral immune suppression
4. Tregs/ T Anergy/ No memory
5. Viral integration; lesion heterogeneity

> ### Box 6.1 Outstanding issues in immune control of HPV associated neoplasia
>
> - What are the key immune mechanisms involved?
>   - i.e. the balance of innate/adaptive immunity.
> - What are the HPV targets?
>   - Many studies have examined responses to E6 and E7, but the other early proteins have been less well studied.
> - What are the kinetics?
>   - Antibodies can be detected in about 50% of women between 4 months and 5 years after exposure but do not necessarily provide protection against new infection. Protection can apparently occur in the absence of antibodies.
>   - T cell responses measured in peripheral blood at low levels may not reflect local activity and are present with progressive disease.
>   - Local immune factors are very difficult to study.
> - What are the genetics?
>   - Immunogenetic factors have been described but are complex and pose far less relative risk compared to persistent high-risk HPV.
> - Is there total protection from infection?
>   - Probably not since naturally induced neutralizing antibodies do not necessarily prevent infection and early episomal infection of stem cells has little viral gene expression.
> - What is the prevalence of latent infection?
>   - Unknown.

and its precise location, as well as a lack of knowledge of the kinetics of integrated viral, tissue, and immune factors. Nevertheless, it will be important to understand whether second or third infections with HPV 16 are new ones or reactivation of previous latent infections. Is there a failure of protective immunity or is it simply not effective enough to provide for total protection? While neutralizing antibodies are generated in many individuals exposed to HPV 16, these may have developed as a consequence of effective activation of cellular immunity, either innate and/or adaptive, and these effector mechanisms may be pivotal in delivering viral clearance with antibodies developing subsequently. Fortunately, in the majority of women, the integrated role of tissue homeostatic, innate, and adaptive immune components successfully clears the HPV virus, which operationally results in the absence of detectable disease. The generation of supranormal levels of neutralizing antibodies by VLP-based vaccines offers exciting prospects for universal prophylactic vaccination (Chapters 7–10). The continuing presence of the viral oncogenes which drive the process of carcinogenesis makes them the prime targets for vaccines aimed at therapy (Chapters 12 and 13).

Further reading

Leggat RG and Frazer IH (2007). HPV vaccines: the beginning of the end for cervical cancer. *Current Opinion in Immunology*, **19**: 232–8.

Moscicki A-B, Schiffman M, Kjaer S, Villa LL (2006). Updating the natural history of HPV and anogenital cancer. *Vaccine*, **24S3**: S3/42–S3/51.

Stanley M (2006). Immune responses to human papilloma virus. *Vaccine*, **24S1**: S1/16–S1/22.

Stern PL (2005). Immune control of human papilloma virus (HPV) associated anogenital disease and potential for vaccination. *Journal of Clinical Virology*, **32S1**: S72–S81.

van der Burg SH, Piersma, SJ, de Jong A, *et al.* (2007). Association of cervical cancer with the presence of CD4-regulatory T cells specific for human papilloma virus antigens. *Proceedings of National Academy of Sciences, USA*, **104**: 12087–92.

Chapter 7

Prophylactic HPV vaccines: pre-clinical and proof of principle studies

Margaret A Stanley

Key points

- Studies of natural papilloma virus infections in the dog, rabbit, and cow showed serum induction of antibody responses to viral capsid proteins. Sero-positive animals were protected for life against challenge with high virus inocula.

- Neutralizing serum antibody responses are directed against the L1 capsid protein. These responses depended on L1 in the native configuration, that is, correctly folded.

- It was shown that the major capsid protein L1 of HPV 16, either with L2 or alone, when expressed via eukaryotic recombinant expression vectors self-assembled into empty protein shells or virus-like particles (VLPs); these were morphologically and antigenically comparable to wild-type papilloma virus virions.

- Rabbits, cows, and dogs immunized with the relevant species-specific VLPs were protected against high-dose viral challenge.

- Proof of principle phase I trials in human subjects showed HPV 16, 11, 6, and 18 VLPs were well tolerated and highly immunogenic, generating HPV L1 type-specific antibody responses at least 100-fold higher than those observed in natural infections with these genital HPV types.

- A proof of principle phase II trial of a monovalent HPV 16 L1 VLP vaccine in HPV 16 naïve women 16–23 years of age demonstrated 100% efficacy against persistent HPV 16 infection and 100% against HPV 16 associated CIN.

7.1 **Background**

It is sobering to reflect that only about 30 years ago human papilloma virus (HPV) were thought to be a small and rather insignificant group of viruses that caused unsightly but trivial excrescences (aka warts) on skin and mucosal surfaces. Since then there has been an explosion of knowledge about these agents, revealing them to be major human pathogens responsible, globally, for significant morbidity and mortality. A small subset of HPVs, particularly HPV 16 and 18, that infect the mucosal surfaces of the ano-genital tract in men and women are true carcinogens—the cause of the majority of cancers of the cervix, 90% or more of anal cancers, at least 40–50% of cancers of the vulva, vagina, and penis, and 10–12% of cancers of the oropharynx. Overall, about 4% of the total global cancer burden can be attributed to the oncogenic high-risk HPVs, particularly HPV 16 (see also Chapters 4 and 10).

In parallel with the molecular and epidemiological studies that confirmed the oncogenicity of the HPVs, there have been efforts focussed on an understanding of the immunobiology of HPV infection and the development of strategies for the prevention and control of this by prophylactic vaccination. The virology and immunology of HPVs is covered in other chapters of this volume (Chapters 3 and 6), but it is worth reiterating some aspects of HPV pathogenesis that made the development of prophylactic vaccines challenging. There are two critical aspects of papilloma virus biology. First, they have an absolutely restricted host range, HPVs infect only humans, dog papilloma viruses infect only dogs and other canines, and so forth. Unfortunately, there is no papilloma virus that infects the laboratory mouse, and experimental studies on pathogenesis had to be restricted to large and relatively expensive animal models of natural infection such as the rabbit, dog, and cow, for which large amounts of infectious virus could be harvested from lesions. Second, HPVs show an exquisite tissue tropism such that only differentiated epithelium will support the complete infectious cycle and the production of infectious particles. Because of this, HPVs cannot be propagated in the amounts needed for vaccines in conventional tissue culture, and few virus particles can be isolated from lesions, effectively preventing the development of conventional live attenuated or dead viral vaccines. The exclusively intra-epithelial replication cycle of the HPVs is one in which the virus makes strenuous efforts to avoid the attention of the immune system; there is no or little viraemia, and infectious virions are shed from mucosal surfaces with poor access to blood, lymph, and draining lymph nodes. As a result, systemic antibody responses to the genital HPVs are slow and weak (the average sero-conversion time for HPV 16 is 8–9 months after the first detection of HPV DNA) and circulating antibody levels are low, all of which might suggest that serum virus neutralizing antibody would not be effective in preventing infection of the epithelial surface. However, in a pioneering study by Shope in the 1930s with the cotton-tail rabbit papilloma virus (CRPV), it was shown that rabbits immunized systemically by intramuscular (i.m.) injection with infectious virus that did not develop visible lesions or papillomas but did develop neutralizing antibodies, and were protected against a cutaneous challenge with large amounts of virus.

7.2 Humoral immunity to papilloma viruses

Subsequent serological studies exploiting natural infections in animals (dog, rabbit, and cow) showed clearly that there were serum responses to viral capsid proteins in individuals who were or had been infected. In the animal models, sero-positive individuals were resistant to subsequent high-dose viral challenge. In early immunization experiments in the rabbit and cow, bacterially expressed L1 and L2 capsid proteins were used as immunogens. In the cow, immunization with BPV-2 L1 protein protected against subsequent viral challenge and prevented papilloma formation. Interestingly, BPV-2 L2 was effective both prophylactically and therapeutically. In the rabbit, immunization with either L1 or L2 protected against CRPV challenge, but L1 was more effective and generated high neutralizing antibody concentrations. Importantly, in these experiments neutralizing antibody was generated only by full-length native L1 protein.

The situation in humans was more challenging, and studies on humoral immunity to HPV, particularly to the high-risk genital HPVs, were seriously hampered since neither clinical lesions nor *in vitro* culture systems were practical sources of virus. It was clear from two specific situations—HPV 1, a virus that could be harvested from plantar warts, and HPV 11 where virions could be generated using an athymic nude mouse xenograft system of HPV 11 infected genital wart tissue—that antibody responses to capsid proteins occurred in infected individuals and that these were to both conformational and linear epitopes. However, the dominant immune response, which was type specific, was to conformational determinants on the intact virus particle and therefore antigen targets in sero-assays and any prophylactic vaccine candidates had to include correctly folded native proteins.

7.3 Generation of virus-like particles (VLPs)

Unfortunately, bacterially expressed fusion proteins of HPV L1 were insoluble and did not assume the native conformation. The challenge was to generate the native correctly folded protein. This challenge was met in a series of seminal studies in the early 1990s, using eukaryotic rather than prokaryotic expression systems. First, using vaccinia virus as an expression system Zhou and Frazer showed that the L1 and L2 capsid proteins of HPV 16 could self-assemble together, generating empty protein capsids (no DNA) or virus-like particles (VLPs). Then it was shown using the baculovirus expression system that the HPV 16 L1 capsid protein alone could self-assemble into VLPs. In both these sets of experiments the yield of VLPs were low, but the HPV 16 L1 gene used to generate the recombinant vectors was cloned from the prototype HPV 16 DNA that had been isolated from a cervical carcinoma in the zur Hausen laboratory in 1983. When L1 cloned from HPV 16, DNA isolated from a low-grade cervical lesion was used to make the recombinant baculovirus, VLP yield was increased fourfold, and it was then shown that the proto-type L1 gene, compared with the wild type L1, had a mutation that affected the efficiency with which VLPs could be assembled. Successful expression and formation of HPV 11 L1 VLPs, using recombinant baculovirus that recognized antibodies in the sera of infected individuals was then demonstrated and it became clear that this was a technology that could be successfully used to generate VLPs of any papilloma virus, including the common genital HPVs (Figure 7.1). L1 VLPs have now been expressed for many different papilloma virus types in a multitude of expression systems, including recombinant vaccinia, baculo- and Semliki Forest virus, yeast VLPs, and plants and can also be generated from bacterially expressed L1 by denaturation/renaturation of the protein under controlled conditions. L1 VLPs lack the minor capsid protein L2 and viral DNA, but are morphologically similar to virions and crucially they closely approximate the antigenic characteristics of wild-type virions.

7.4 **Sero-epidemiologic studies using HPV L1 VLPs**

L1 VLPs were and continue to be used extensively in sero-epidemiological studies in humans, revealing that type-specific antibody responses are common during and after infection with genital HPVs. About 50–60% of women currently infected with HPV 16 (as measured by PCR positivity in cervical swabs or washings) have serum antibodies reactive with HPV 16 VLPs. Prospective studies indicate that 70–90% of women seroconvert with a mean time of 8 months elapsing between acquisition of HPV DNA and seroconversion. Several studies have shown that sero-positivity to capsid proteins is associated with increasing severity of CIN but decreases in patients with invasive carcinoma. Seropositivity to HPV 16 VLPs is associated with an increased risk for the development of cervical carcinoma,

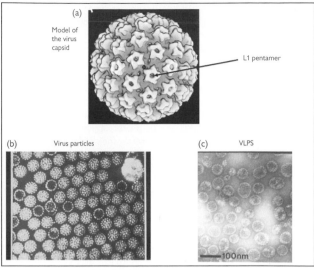

Figure 7.1 (a) A model of the papilloma virus capsid. The rosette-like surface structures (arrowed) are pentamers each consisting of five molecules of L1; one molecule of L2 fits into the central dimple of each pentamer. (b) Papilloma virus particles; both full (contain DNA) and empty particles can be seen. (c) HPV 16 L1 virus-like particles made by expressing HPV 16 L1 in baculovirus. The L1 protein thus expressed spontaneously assembles into empty capsids or VLPs that are morphologically similar to the empty virus particles seen in panel (b). Reproduced from Stanley M, DR Lowy, I Frazer. Chapter 12: Prophylactic HPV vaccines: underlying mechanisms. *Vaccine*, 2006; **24**(Suppl 3): S106–13 with permission from Elsevier.

supporting the notion that viral persistence is a key factor in disease progression in the cervix. Overall, the evidence from studies on both the high- and low-risk genital viruses is that specific antibody responses to the L1 capsid protein as measured in the VLP ELISA (enzyme-linked immunsorbent assay) are common during, and after, infection with genital HPVs. The low sensitivity of the assay and the variability of the interval between infection and seroconversion suggest that serum antibody responses would not be useful for diagnosis in the individual patient.

7.5 **VLP vaccines: animal models**

These data suggested that VLPs that generated neutralizing antibody to HPV L1 would be effective in prophylaxis, and experimental studies that show immunogenicity and efficacy with L1 VLP vaccines in three animal models—the dog, cow, and rabbit—supported this notion. In these three species (dog, cow, and rabbit) immunization with

COPV, BPV, or CRPV L1 VLPs induced circulating, neutralizing antibody to the L1 capsid protein, and the immunized animals were completely resistant to challenge with high virus inocula. Importantly, in the rabbit model relatively long-term protection was induced by VLP immunization. The data from the dog are particularly relevant for genital HPVs, since the COPV is a mucosatrophic virus infecting the oral cavity. Conformational epitopes on intact VLPs are immunodominant and appear critical for the induction of neutralizing IgG and for successful vaccination, since denatured COPV L1 protein fails to generate neutralizing antibody or protect against virus challenge; but formaldehyde-fixed COPV VLPs retain their immunogenicity and protect against virus. Irrespective of the expression system used, immunization with the species-specific L1 prior to virus challenge has been shown to be protective in all the animal models tested. Immunization with a DNA polynucleotide vaccine encoding the L1 gene was successful in both the rabbit and the dog protecting against virus challenge and a COPV L1 expressing recombinant adenovirus protected in the dog.

In the animal models, successful immunization was species specific and mediated by serum antibody. In rabbits, passive transfer of serum or purified IgG from hyperimmune animals immunized with CRPV L1/L2 VLPs completely protected the naïve recipients from challenge with 10^{10} infectious virus particles. Of the four animals challenged with 10^{11} virus particles, three developed small papillomas that rapidly regressed. Twelve-week old beagle dogs, shown to be negative for maternal antibody to COPV, were immunized with purified IgG or total immune IgG derived from immune serum of dogs in which COPV-induced papillomas had spontaneously regressed. The animals immunized with anti-COPV L1 IgG were completely protected from challenge with high levels of virus. These studies demonstrate that serum IgG conferred protection and the most likely explanation is that this was mediated via serum neutralizing IgG. However, it should be noted that although there is no doubt that protection was via serum IgG in these experiments, the evidence that neutralizing IgG mediated the effect was indirect in both. Nonetheless, the data overall consistently show that L1 VLPs induce high levels of serum neutralizing IgG, and the results of VLP vaccination both in animal infections and clinical trials support the notion that it is this activity that is critical for protection. The role of local mucosal antibody remains unclear. Cervico-vaginal lavage fluid harvested from immunized primates neutralizes HPV 11 particles, but only 50% of women immunised with HPV 11 L1 VLPs were shown to develop local mucosal anti-HPV antibody. IgG is the principal immunoglobulin in cervical secretions and the assumption, at the present, is that VLP vaccine-induced protection is mediated by serum IgG (predominantly neutralizing IgG) that can transudate across the basement membrane of the cervical epithelium, particularly at the squamo-columnar junction, in high enough concentration to bind to virus particles, thus preventing infection.

7.6 VLP vaccines: proof of principle immunogenicity and safety studies in human subjects

L1 VLPs were clearly candidate immunogens for prophylactic vaccination in humans, and randomized double blind placebo-controlled phase I studies with recombinant HPV L1 VLP vaccines were undertaken to show immunogenicity and safety. These showed that all VLP-immunized subjects, but no subjects in the placebo arms, sero-converted and made anti-VLP antibody responses substantially greater than that identified in natural infections. In most studies, the vaccine was delivered with an aluminium hydroxide or a proprietary aluminium hydroxyphosphate sulphate adjuvant; but Harro and colleagues in 2001 looked at responses without adjuvant in comparison with those with alum or MF59 (an oil and water emulsion) as adjuvant. Antibody responses were dose dependent when vaccine was given without adjuvant or with MF59 but were dose independent when administered with alum. The dominant antibody response was of the IgG1 subclass and was shown to be neutralizing by an HPV 16 pseudovirion neutralizing assay. In a phase I, blinded, placebo-controlled, randomized dose escalation study of baculovirus expressed HPV 11 L1 VLPs, anti-VLP neutralizing antibodies were induced that declined by about fivefold between weeks 20 and 48 post-vaccination. Overall the data from published phase I studies using HPV VLP vaccines including HPV 16 or 18 and/or HPV 6/11 L1 VLPs showed that the HPV VLP vaccines were safe, well tolerated, and highly immunogenic, inducing high levels of both binding- and neutralizing-type antibodies.

7.7 Proof of principle efficacy study with a monovalent HPV 16 L1 VLP vaccine

The efficacy of a monovalent HPV 16 vaccine was assessed in a double blind, placebo-controlled, proof of principle study reported by Koutsky and others in 2002. In this seminal study 2392 women aged between 16 and 23 were randomized to receive vaccine (3 doses of 40mcg of yeast-derived HPV 16 VLP adjuvanted with aluminium hydroxy-phosphate sulphate at 0, 2, and 6 months) or adjuvant alone as a placebo. The primary endpoint of the trial was detection of persistent cervico-vaginal HPV 16 infection where this was defined as HPV 16 DNA detected in consecutive samples (obtained at consecutive visits 6 months or more apart) using a sensitive type-specific PCR for HPV 16 or 18. The results of this study were stunning. Of the 1533 individuals naïve at entry for HPV 16 DNA followed for a median of 17 months, HPV 16 DNA was detected in none of the vaccinees compared with 41 of the placebo group, 9 of whom had HPV-related CIN grades I or II. Although this study was not powered for efficacy against HPV 16 associated CIN, no cases of CIN of any grade were found in the vaccine group compared with nine cases in the placebo group, of which one case was a CIN2. Follow-up on this trial cohort was maintained and at 48 months after the initial immunization vaccine, efficacy remained at 100% for HPV 16 positive CIN of any grade in the 755 women who had received the HPV 16 L1 VLP vaccine. HPV 16 specific serum antibody titres were measured using radioimmunoassay; peak antibody concentrations were achieved 1 month after the third immunization, antibody concentrations waned over the following 12 months and then plateaued, and were maintained at levels 8- to 10-fold those achieved in natural infections up to 48 months after the initial immunization.

7.8 **Conclusion**

The development of HPV prophylactic vaccines targeting the two most important oncogenic HPV types, 16 and 18, is a major achievement for biomedical research and development. The route from bench to clinic for any new vaccine or drug is usually long and often difficult, but for HPV vaccines it has been relatively short—11 years between the laboratory generation of VLPs to publication of the proof of principle efficacy trial. These vaccines illustrate with great clarity the power of modern molecular techniques and are truly vaccines for the 21st century with the promise that if effectively implemented they will prevent the majority of cervical cancers worldwide.

Further reading

Breitburd F, Kirnbauer R, Hubbert NL, et al. (1995). Immunization with virus-like particles from cotton tail rabbit papilloma virus (CRPV) can protect against experimentally CRPV infection. *Journal of Virology*, **69**: 3959–63.

Evans TG, Bonnez W, Rose RC, Koenig S, et al. (2001). A Phase 1 study of a recombinant virus like particle vaccine against human papilloma virus type 11 in healthy adult volunteers. *Journal of Infectious Disease*, **183**: 1485–93.

Harro CD, Pang YY, Roden RB, *et al.* (2001). Safety and immunogenicity trial in adult volunteers of a human papilloma virus 16 L1 virus-like particle vaccine. *Journal of National Cancer Institute*, **93**: 284–92.

Kirnbauer R, Booy F, Cheng N, *et al.* (1992). Papilloma virus L1 major capsid protein self-assembles into virus-like particles that are highly immunogenic. Proceedings of the National Academy of Science, USA, **89**: 12180–4.

Koutsky LA, Ault KA, Wheeler CM, *et al.* (2002). A controlled trial of a human papilloma virus type 16 vaccine. *New England Journal of Medicine*, **347**: 1645–51.

Stanley MA (2006). HPV vaccines. In A. Fiander, ed. Best practice in obstetrics and gynaecology: gynaecological cancer screening and prevention, **20**: 279–93.

Suzich JA, Ghim SJ, Palmer Hill, FJ, *et al.* (1995). Systemic immunization with papilloma virus L1 protein completely prevents the development of viral mucosal papillomas. *Proceedings of the National Academy of Sciences, USA,* **92**: 11553–7.

Zhou J, Sun XY, Stenzel DJ, *et al.* (1991). Expression of vaccinia recombinant HPV 16 L1 and L2 ORF proteins in epithelial cells is sufficient for assembly of HPV virion like particles. *Virology*, **185**: 251–7.

Chapter 8

Prophylactic HPV vaccination: current status

Henry C Kitchener

Key points

- Prophylactic human papilloma virus (HPV) vaccines have been developed against types 16 and 18, based on virus-like particles (VLPs) and which induce high titres of neutralizing antibodies, could potentially prevent 70% of cancers worldwide.
- These vaccines are more than 90% effective at preventing type 16/18 associated CIN, although overall efficacy against all type CIN2/3 in all vaccine recipients, irrespective of current infection is considerably less.
- There is evidence that the bivalent vaccine provides significant cross protection against CIN2+ associated with types 31, 33 and 45 and the quadrivalent vaccine against CIN 2+ associated with type 31.
- The quadrivalent vaccine has shown efficacy against type 16/18 related CIN2+ in women aged 24-45 who do not have 16/18 infection.
- The optimal age group to vaccinate is pre-adolescent girls.
- The possible need for booster vaccination to maintain protection can only be determined by further follow-up data.

8.1 Introduction

Enormous public interest has been generated over the last year with the licensing of two vaccines designed to prevent human papilloma virus (HPV) cancer of the cervix. In Chapter 7, the development of these vaccines was described together with proof of principle. In this chapter, the results of recently published clinical trials will be reviewed and the implications discussed.

The rationale of prophylactic HPV vaccination is based on the necessity of HPV infection in cervical carcinogenesis, so that by preventing this primary event, secondary changes which result in cytological abnormalities will also be prevented. It is the prevention of pathological change in the cervix which is the purpose of the vaccine, because the infection itself is asymptomatic and does not cause acute damage. This concept of preventing a viral infection to prevent a cancer, which might otherwise not occur for 25 years, is novel and differs from the usual role of vaccines, which is to prevent an infection that causes acute morbidity. Perhaps hepatitis B is the closest model where the vaccine is designed to prevent not only an acute infection but also chronic disease in which state carriers can not only be highly infectious but can also sustain serious liver damage. Furthermore, susceptible populations have a high risk of developing liver cancer, and falling rates of hepatocellular cancer are now being seen in vaccinated populations in the Far East.

In many developed countries, a strategy of secondary prevention of cervical cancer is employed through well-established cervical screening programmes (CSPs) (see Chapter 1). A strategy of primary prevention would reduce the amount of morbidity associated with the management of abnormal cytology, and would also offer a potential means of prevention in countries without any cervical screening which includes many underdeveloped countries with high rates of cervical cancer.

8.2 **HPV infection**

In order to use the vaccine most effectively, it is necessary to understand the natural history of HPV infection. This occurs most frequently following the onset of sexual activity which is widespread among UK teenagers from the age of 15, although it is recognized that a significant proportion of younger girls are sexually active from 14 years. It is also quite clear that the acquisition of HPV infection is fairly rapid such that 50% of adolescents will acquire HPV within 2–3 years (recently reviewed by Moscicki 2007). Most cervical infections clear spontaneously within 12 months, but in around 40% of cases the virus will persist in the cervix for over a year and in some cases longer (Kjaer et al. 2002), which increases the risk of cervical intraepithelial neoplasia (CIN) developing in future years.

As outlined in Chapter 4, there are around 15 HPV types which are associated with cervical cancer worldwide, and although HPV 16 is by far the most prevalent type seen in the late stages of cervical carcinogenesis, in low-grade abnormalities other types are almost as prevalent. As shown in Table 8.1, unless type-specific vaccines crossprotect against other types, many low-grade lesions would not be prevented (Kitchener et al. 2006). Genital warts, which are caused mainly by HPV 6 and most commonly seen on the vulva, constitute a major public health issue although these do not predispose to cervical cancer.

Table 8.1 Prevalence of HPV 16, HPV 18, and other high-risk HPV types by age, cytology, and histology at entry

Age	HC-II negatives	HPV 16	HPV 18 (not HPV 16)	Other HC-II positives*	Total
20–24	1548 (60.1%)	315 (12.2%)	80 (3.1%)	632 (24.6%)	2575 (100%)
25–34	4867 (77.6%)	320 (5.1%)	127 (2.0%)	957 (15.3%)	6271 (100%)
25–34	6538 (89.2%)	112 (1.5%)	43 (0.6%)	638 (8.7%)	7331 (100%)
45–54	4707 (92.2%)	35 (0.7%)	15 (03.%)	345 (6.8%)	5102 (100%)
55–64	3037 (94.0%)	21 (0.7%)	7 (0.2%)	166 (5.1%)	3231 (100%)
Cytology					
Normal	19 154 (89.6%)	318 (1.5%)	143 (0.7%)	1765 (8.2%)	21 380 (100%)
Borderline	1232 (68.9%)	125 (7.0%)	54 (3.0%)	378 (21.1%)	1789 (100%)
Mild	265 (30.2%)	152 (17.3%)	40 (4.6%)	421 (47.9%)	878 (100%)
Moderate	38 (14.0%)	107 (39.5%)	18 (6.6%)	108 (39.9%)	271 (100%)
Severe or worse	8 (4.2%)	101 (52.6%)	17 (8.8%)	66 (34.4%)	192 (100%)
Histology					
CINI or less	318 (40.8%)	104 (13.3%)	48 (6.2%)	310 (39.7%)	780 (100%)
CIN2	15 (7.1%)	85 (40.1%)	15 (7.1%)	97 (45.7%)	212 (100%)
CIN3/SCC	7 (2.7%)	157 (60.4%)	14 (5.4%)	82 (31.5%)	260 (100%)
CGIN/ADC	3 (16.7%)	6 (33.3%)	6 (33.3%)	3 (16.7%)	18 (100%)
Abnormal cytology, no histology	1200 (64.5%)	133 (7.1%)	45 (2.5%)	481 (25.9%)	1860 (100%)
Total	20 697 (84.4%)	803 (3.3%)	272 (1.1%)	2738 (11.2%)	24 510 (100%)

SCC: Squamous cell carcinoma; CGIN: Cervical glandular intraepithelial neoplasia; ADC: Adenocarcinoma.

* Not HPV 16 or HPV 18;

** Women with abnormal cytology at entry but no histology (abnormal cytology resolved or still being followed-up cytologically).

Source: Taken from Kitchener et al. British Journal of Cancer, 2006.

8.3 **The vaccines**

The principle of prophylactic vaccination to prevent cervical cancer relies on the generation of neutralizing antibodies, which prevent subsequent infection with high-risk types of HPV. Virus-like particles (VLPs) that structurally mimic the native virions can be produced by expressing the HPV type-specific L1 proteins, using recombinant yeast or baculoviral technologies (Chapter 7). Currently, two licensed prophylactic vaccines have been developed and tested in large randomized trials. The first of these is a quadrivalent vaccine directed against types 6, 11, 16, and 18, known as Gardasil® which is manufactured in yeast and uses an aluminium adjuvant and is designed to prevent genital warts as well as cervical cancer. The second is a bivalent vaccine directed against types 16 and 18 which is known as Cervarix® and incorporates a novel adjuvant, ASO4. Table 8.2 summarizes some key properties of the two vaccines and their recommended uses. In both cases the vaccine had been previously tested in randomized phase II studies which confirmed both immunogenicity and prevention of incident and persistent type-specific infection. As described in Chapter 4, these vaccines are expected to be capable of preventing 70% of cervical cancer in any fully vaccinated population. From the perspective of an individual, the vaccine would reduce that woman's risk of developing abnormal cytology and cancer. As will be seen later, the degree of protection depends on prior exposure to HPV.

8.4 **The clinical trials**

Both vaccines have been tested in large randomized phase II trials and subsequently in pivotal phase III trials, one of which has published final results and the other the results of an interim analysis. The phase II studies were designed to confirm sustained immunogenicity and some evidence of efficacy relevant to definitive endpoints of a pivotal efficacy trial. The phase III trials were designed to demonstrate the level of conclusive evidence of efficacy required to obtain a marketing licence and convince funders that the vaccine is sufficiently effective and cost effective for public health programmes. This requires evidence of the prevention of CIN3 as a surrogate for cancer prevention.

In Chapter 7, the first trial data to confirm the proof of principle with regard to the potential role of VLP vaccine was presented (Koutsky et al. 2002). In this chapter, more mature data from each of the phase II trials together with the most recently published data from the phase III trials will be presented and discussed in terms of public health benefit.

Table 8.2 Vaccine properties and uses*

	CERVARIX	GARDASIL
Clinical effectiveness	Prevention of high-grade CIN2/3 and cervical cancer causally related to HPV types 16 and 18 in girls/women aged 10–25 based on efficacy data in 15- to 25-year-old women, as well as bridging immunogenicity studies in 10 to 14-year-old girls and boys.	Prevention of high-grade CIN2/3, cervical, high-grade VIN2/3, and genital warts causally related to HPV types 6/11/6 and 18 in girls/women aged 9–26 years based on efficacy studies in women 15–26 as well as bridging studies demonstrating immunogenicity in girls and boys aged 9–15
Active ingredients	Each dose HPV 16 L1 protein (20mcg) HPV 18 L1 protein (20mcg)	Each dose: HPV 6 L1 protein (20mcg), HPV 11 L1 protein (40mcg), HPV 16 L1 protein (40mcg) HPV 18 L1 Protein (20mcg)
Adjuvant	ASO4—monophosphoryl lipid A adsorbed on aluminium hydroxide	Alum—amorphous aluminium hydroxy-phosphate sulphate
Dosage and schedule	One 0.5ml dose at 0, 1, and 6 months by IM injection in the deltoid region	One 0.5ml dose at 0, 2, and 6 months by IM injection in the deltoid or anterolateral thigh
Side effects**		
Very common	Injection site reactions, headache, myalgia	Injection site reactions, fever
Common	Gastrointestinal symptoms, itching/pruritus/ rash urticaria, arthralgia, and fever ≥38°C	Bleeding, itching at the site of injection
Uncommon	Dizziness, URTI, injection site induration/paraesthesia	Urticaria bronchospam

Common properties: Store at 2–8°C, do not freeze. Not for SC/IV administration. No data in subjects with impaired immune responsiveness, postpone until after pregnancy, may be administered to lactating women.

Source: Adapted from *British Medical Journal* online Tristram, Daayana, and Stern 2008.

* This is not prescribing information.

** A full list of side effects is supplied with product information

Before the trial data are presented, it is necessary to consider different categories of participant data that are described in these studies. This is because the women who have been recruited to these trials will receive varying degrees of protection from a prophylactic vaccine according to whether they have already been exposed to a genital infection, whether they sero-converted, and whether they received the full regimen of vaccine. In terms of proof of principle, individuals who are HPV positive at the time of vaccination or who do not receive the full regimen of vaccine can legitimately be excluded from the analysis. When it comes to definitive efficacy studies all of the data need to be included in the primary analysis if the generalizable efficacy of the vaccine for the population in the trial is to be determined. It is, however, necessary to divide the results into data from different categories of participants if the true level of protection which the vaccine is capable of providing is to be determined. So, for example, quite clearly a 12-year-old, non-HPV exposed virgin, is more likely to be protected from a type-specific HPV infection than a 16-year-old who has had more than one sexual partner and who was HPV positive prior to receiving the vaccine. It is also necessary to separate HPV-related outcomes into the types specific to the vaccine and other types against which the vaccine may or may not protect. This is particularly important because there is a broad range of virus types capable of causing lesions relevant to the outcomes in these trials.

The following terms will be used and are derived from the original publications:

- 'Per-protocol susceptible', meaning recipients who were HPV DNA negative on cervical testing and seronegative prior to vaccination, and who received three doses of vaccine with no protocol violation. These individuals would also remain DNA negative throughout the vaccination period. The relevant outcome is type 16/18 CIN2+ positivity.
- 'Unrestricted susceptible', meaning HPV DNA negative and seronegative prior to vaccination but with imperfect compliance, for example, not receiving three doses of vaccine. Again type 16/18 CIN2+ positivity is the relevant outcome.
- 'Intention to treat', meaning all randomized subjects irrespective of HPV status and compliance. All type associated CIN as well as type 16/18 CIN is the relevant outcome.

8.4.1 Trial # 1: Prophylactic quadrivalent human papilloma virus (types 6, 11, 16, 18) L1 virus-like particle vaccine in young women: a randomized double blind placebo-controlled multicentre phase II efficacy trial (Villa et al. 2005)

In this study, 227 randomized women received vaccine (20mcg type 6, 40mcg type 11, 40mcg type 16, and 20mcg type 18) and 275 randomized women received placebo. The vaccine contained aluminium adjuvant that was also contained in the placebo preparation. Vaccine was given at 0, 2, and 6 months. Women were aged between

16 and 23 (mean age 20 years) and all but 6% had had at least one sexual partner. The per protocol analysis included 404(73%) for type 16 associated events, 456(83%) for type 18 and 431(78%) for types 6/11.

Only types 6-, 11-, 16-, and 18-related events were reported. There were 36 infection- or disease-related events reported (35 infections/6 disease) in the placebo group and 4 (4 infection/no disease) in the vaccinated group, giving an efficacy difference of 90% (95%CI, 71–97) in the per-protocol group and a similar number in the intention to treat group due to the small numbers.

Immunogenicity was reported which showed that mean antibody titres were 10- to 100-fold higher in the vaccine group compared with the placebo group at 7 months, and although the titres dropped with time at 36 months they remained higher, particularly for type 16 which remained 30-fold higher.

The vaccine was associated with only 1% serious adverse events. Around 80% of both vaccine and placebo recipients experienced injection site pain and around 30–40% experienced systemic effects, usually mild headache.

These results clearly demonstrated the potential of this vaccine, which then underwent assessment in a large international randomized phase III trial (Trial # 3).

8.4.2 Trial # 2: A randomized phase II trial of a bivalent L1 virus-like particle vaccine against human papilloma virus types 16 and 18 (Harper et al. 2004)

In this trial, 560 randomized women received vaccine and 553 randomized women received placebo. The vaccine contained 20mcg each of HPV 16 and 18 with an adjuvant, ASO4, that contained 500mcg aluminium hydroxide and 50mcg 3-deacylated monophosphoryl lipid A. The placebo contained 500mcg aluminium hydroxide. Three doses were given at 0, 1, and 6 months.

The vaccine efficacy in preventing persistent HPV 16/18 specific infection was 91.6% in the per-protocol analysis, with clear evidence of preventing over 90% of cytological abnormalities associated with 16/18. The vaccine was very safe and immunogenic.

This trial subsequently reported follow-up data including long-term efficacy and sustained immunogenicity (Harper et al. 2006). This extended follow-up study reported on 393 vaccine and 383 placebo recipients with a mean follow-up of 47 months. This allowed an analysis with more events and immunogenicity over a longer period. In a per-protocol analysis, vaccinated women experienced 96% protection from persistent type 16 and 18 infection compared with placebo recipients, and similar protection against developing types 16 and 18 associated cytological abnormality (ASCUS+). This level of protection fell to 48% when all cytological abnormalities, irrespective of HPV type, were considered.

With regard to immunogenicity, there was clear evidence of sustained antibody with titres being maintained at levels around 100-fold that in the placebo group. Evidence of cross-protection against non 16/18 high-risk types would be important because if this extended to clinically relevant outcomes it would add breadth to the range of prevention offered by the vaccine. In this extended follow-up study, there were data that indicated a virtual absence of incident HPV 45 infection in the vaccinated group (1 vs 17 in the placebo group) and a 50% level of protection against HPV 31 (14 vs 30). This is feasible given that types 16 and 18 are phylogenetically linked to types 31 and 45, respectively. It will require data from large phase III trials to confirm these observations.

These phase II trials indicated convincingly that these vaccines were immunogenic, that the immunogenicity was sustained, and that they protected against type-specific infection with some evidence of cross-protection against types 31 and 45 by the bivalent vaccine. There was early evidence of protection against CIN2/3, but these trials were not powered to show efficacy against cancer precursor lesions. To provide convincing evidence of a public health benefit in terms of the prevention of cervical cancer, it would be necessary to demonstrate a very high level of protection against the widely accepted surrogate lesion, CIN 3, or at least CIN 2/3. To achieve this within a relatively short timescale, large trials were required.

8.4.3 Trial # 3: A phase III randomized trial of a quadrivalent vaccine against human papilloma virus to prevent high-grade cervical lesions (FUTURE II study group 2007)

This was the first large international pivotal trial to report on the efficacy of a VLP vaccine in the prevention of high-grade CIN. The trial known as FUTURE II opened in June 2002, recruited 12 167 women over a period of 12 months, and reported in May 2007. The vaccine used and the regimen were the same as that described in Trial #1. The study population comprised females aged 15–26 (mean age 20) recruited in 90 centres in 13 countries. The population included 948 and 397 women were either seropositive or DNA positive in the cervix for types 16 and 18, respectively.

An earlier interim analysis had been performed as part of the licensure application to the Food and Drug Administration (FDA); this report was the final analysis of the primary endpoint, type 16 or 18 specific CIN2 or worse, which required at least 29 events. In the final analysis there was a total of 43 type 16-/18-specific CIN2+ lesions in the total per-protocol susceptible population (10 565), 65 in the unrestricted susceptible population (11 728), and 485 in the intention to treat population (12 167).

The vaccine efficacy against type 16-/18-specific CIN2+ in the per-protocol susceptible population was 98% (95% CI 86–100). This approximates to what could be expected amongst a sexually naïve population of young adolescents who had received all three doses of the vaccine. Amongst the unrestricted but susceptible population the efficacy against type 16-/18-specific lesions was similar, 95% (95% CI 85–99). When all randomized vaccinated subjects were included, that is, the intention to treat population, the overall vaccine efficacy for 16-/18-type specific CIN2+ was 44%. This represents the 'real-life' estimate of prevention in an unselected population of women in this age group. Although type 16-associated CIN may be more likely to progress to cancer if untreated, all CIN are regarded as requiring treatment and, therefore, the intention to treat analysis for CIN of any HPV type represents the true test of efficacy in terms of disease prevention. The vaccine efficacy in this setting was 17% (95% CI 1–31).

The explanation for this range of efficacy lies both in the fact that in this population a significant proportion of women were already HPV 16/18 positive and also that high-grade CIN is associated with a range of HPV high-risk types. Data published from the ARTISTIC trial demonstrated that only around half of high-grade cytology was associated with HPV types 16 and 18 (Kitchener et al. 2006).

One of the key attributes of the quadrivalent vaccine is the inclusion of types 6 and 11 designed to protect against genital warts. In a second paper from a different study population (Garland et al. 2007) data were presented for both condylomata (warts) arising in the vulva and vagina, and for vulval/vaginal intraepithelial neoplasia (VIN/VAIN). In this study known as FUTURE I, which ran contemporaneously with the FUTURE II study, 5455 women aged between 16 and 24 years were randomly assigned to receive the same vaccine or placebo.

In terms of vaccine efficacy against genital warts, the vaccine was highly protective. The per-protocol, unrestricted susceptible, and intention to treat analyses demonstrated efficacy of 100% (95% CI 94–100), 96% (95% CI 86–99), and 76% (95% CI 61–86), respectively.

Type 16-/18-specific VIN and VAIN grades 2/3 have also been reported in a recent paper (Joura et al. 2007) combining the data from the FUTURE I and II studies to increase the numbers. The reported efficacy for type 16-/18-specific VIN/VAIN grades 2/3 was 100% (15 cases vs 0) and 49% (53 cases vs 27) for all type lesions, by intention to treat.

Early data presented by the FUTURE Group indicated some cross-protection against CIN associated with types 31/33/45 combined (Brown et al. 2007). More recent data have established that there is only significant cross protection against type 31 CIN or adenocarcinoma in situ with an efficacy of 56.9% (C.I. 28.6-74.8%) and no demonstrable protection against type 33 or 45 (Brown et al 2009).

The results from the FUTURE I and II studies are summarized in Table 8.3 together with those from the PATRICIA study (see Section 8.4.4).

Table 8.3 Summary of HVP VLP Vaccine Efficacy Data

Trial	Analysis	No. of randomised subjects	End point	Total no. of cases (vaccine)	Vaccine efficacy % (95% CI)
Future II* adjuvanted (alum) quadrivalent (6, 11, 16, 18) vs adjuvant (placebo) (Gardasil®)	per-protocol (16, 18)	10565	CIN2+	43(1)	98(86–100)
	unrestricted susceptible (16, 18)	11728	CIN2+	65(3)	95(85–99)
	intention to treat (16, 18)	12167	CIN2+	209(77)	42(22–56)
	all types	12167	CIN2+	485(219)	17(1–31)
PATRICIA** Adjuvanted (ASO4) bivalent 16, 18 vs HepA (control)	TVC	18644			
	Per protocol TVC eligible for primary analysis HPV −ve/sero −ve at month 0	14656	CIN2+(16/18)	56(4)	92.9(79.9–98.3)†
	TVC-naïve	10885	CIN2+(16/18)	63(1)	98.4(90.4–100)
			CIN2+ (any HPV)	110(33)	70.2(54.7–80.9)
Future I*** adjuvanted (alum) quadrivalent (6, 11, 16, 18) vs adjuvant (placebo)	per-protocol 6, 11, 16, 18	4540	VIN2+/VAIN2+	9(0)	100(49–100)
		4540	genital warts	48(0)	100(92–100)
	unrestricted susceptible 6, 11, 16, 18	5351	VIN2+/VAIN2+	12(1)	91(31–100)
		5351	genital warts	70(3)	96(86–99)
	intention to treat 6, 11, 16, 18	5455	VIN2/VAIN2	18(5)	62(<0–89)
		5455	genital warts	107(21)	76(61–89)

* Future II Study Group 2007
** Paavonen et al. 2009
*** Garland et al 2007
† 98.1% (C.I. 88.4–100%) in an analysis in which probable causality to HPV type was assigned in lesions with multiple oncogenic infections.

8.4.4 **Trial #4: Efficacy of a prophylactic adjuvanted VLP vaccine against cervical infection and pre-cancer caused by oncogenic HPV types; a final analysis (Paavonen et al, 2009).**

This trial, known as PATRICIA, is the second largest international pivotal trial for which a final analysis has recently been reported. In this trial, 18,644 women aged between 15–25 years were recruited between May 2004 and June 2005 from 14 countries; one third from the Americas, one third from Europe and one third from Asia Pacific countries. The vaccine and regimen used were the same as reported in Trial #2. Among the study population, 80% had negative cytology of whom 15% were high risk HPV DNA positive and 5% HPV16/18 positive. Among women who had high or low grade cytological abnormalities, the HPV 16/18 DNA positive rate was 56% and 29% respectively. Eighty one percent of the study population was both seronegative and DNA negative for type 16 and 87% for type 18.

At the time of reporting mean follow-up was 35 months after the third dose of vaccine. Vaccine efficacy against CIN2+ associated with HPV 16/18 in the per protocol analysis was 92.9% (C.I. 79.9–98.3%) . This was 98.1% (C.I. 88.4–100%) in an analysis in which probable causality to HPV type was assigned in lesions with multiple oncogenic infections. Amongst the total vaccinated cohort (TVC) who were DNA negative for high risk types and seronegative for vaccine types (TVC-naïve which approximates target population being vaccinated in the UK), vaccine efficacy was 70.2% (C.I. 54.7–80.9%). This latter proportion is greater than expected for CIN2+ directly related only to types 16 and 18 and strongly suggests there is cross protection against other types. Additional data presented in a web appendix indicates that in the HPV DNA negative TVC, vaccine efficacy against CIN2+ associated with types 31, 33 and 45 was 68.4%(C.I. 34.2–86.1%), 49.8%(C.I. 4.8–74.6%) and 100% (C.I. 7–100%) respectively.

It is clear that the bivalent vaccine not only achieves a high efficacy against type 16/18 related disease but also against a broader range of CIN2+ lesions. This could translate into 80% protection against cervical cancer.

8.4.5 **Trial #5: A randomised trial of a quadrivalent vaccine against HPV infection and related CIN2+ in women aged 24–45 years (Munoz et al 2009).**

This recently reported randomised trial was the first to report prophylactic vaccine efficacy in women over 25 years. In this study 3,817 women aged 24-45 were randomised to either alum adjuvanted quadrivalent vaccine, directed against HPV 6, 11, 16 and 18, or alum adjuvant alone. Women were accrued between June 2004–May 2005 in North America, Latin America, Asia and Europe. The median age at accrual was 35 years and the majority were using contraception.

One third were seropositive to a vaccine HPV type and 7.9% showed a vaccine HPV type cervical infection at baseline. Ninety percent of the women were PCR negative to 3 or 4 of the vaccine HPV types. Almost all had been sexually active. Vaccine induced antibody titres to the vaccine types were similar across the age range. Titres to type 16 were similar to those seen in 16-23 year olds and were slightly lower for type 6, 11 and 18 in this older cohort.

Vaccine efficacy was reported for persistent infection and CIN combined. In the per protocol population the efficacy against 6, 11, 16, 18 related conditions was 90.5% (C.I. 73.7%–97.5%) based on four cases in the vaccine group and 41 in the placebo. Vaccine efficacy against 16, 18 related conditions was 83.1% (C.I. 50.6%–95.8%) based on four cases in the vaccine group and 23 in the placebo group. The majority of these cases were infection rather then CIN. In the naïve or susceptible group (PCR negative and received at least one dose of vaccine) vaccine efficacy against 6, 11, 18 and 18 conditions was 74.6% and 71.6% against 16 and 18 related conditions. Efficacy was a little less but not significantly so when 24-34 year olds were compared with 35-45 year olds. As expected from previously reported, an intention to treat analysis for all HPV type related conditions indicated much lower efficacy of around 30%.

These results indicate that the quadrivalent vaccine is protective in older women but the data are based on very few cases of CIN and larger trial numbers with longer follow-up will be required to provide convincing evidence of the degree of protection afforded to women in this age range.

8.5 Discussion

The principal findings from these trials are that the VLP vaccines are highly effective at preventing type 16-/18-specific lower genital tract neoplasia, that the quadrivalent vaccine prevents genital warts, and that the vaccines appear safe and free of concern in relation to pregnancy. It is also quite clear that the level of protection afforded by these vaccines depends on the likelihood of having had a previous type 16 or 18 infection. Despite the ability of the vaccines to prevent type-specific CIN, many CIN lesions are associated with other types and this is reflected in the relatively low impact seen for all types of intraepithelial neoplasia in an unselected population. The impact of preventing cancer by preventing type 16-associated disease will be proportionately stronger. Two important recent reports have indicated significant efficacy by the bivalent vaccine to prevent CIN2+ associated with types 31, 33 and 45, while the quadrivalent vaccine achieves high efficacy in preventing 16/18 related CIN2+ in women aged 24-45, provided they do not show 16/18 infection at the time of vaccination.

These vaccines have been licensed in Europe to prevent CIN in all females aged from 9 to 25. Much consideration has been given and continues to be given by government and other funders to the provision of these vaccines to susceptible populations. In some countries, vaccination is to be made available free of charge to young adolescent girls aged 10–13, and in some countries a so-called catch-up programme of older adolescents will be offered. In the United Kingdom, the Departments of Health have implemented a national programme for 12- and 13-year-olds during the school year beginning in 2008. Catch-up vaccination on girls up to the age of 18 will be phased over 3 years, so by 2011 all UK females 18 years old and younger will have been offered vaccination. Vaccination of boys is not being seriously considered at the moment because evidence regarding its effectiveness is lacking, and penile cancer is rare.

There are a number of other key issues to be considered in the implementation of vaccination and these will be considered in ensuing chapters. These include the following:

- The implications for cervical screening in the presence of a vaccination programme
- The development of vaccines with a broader reach in terms of type-specific infection notwithstanding any cross-protection afforded by the current vaccines
- The importance of developing public confidence in the vaccines and getting a sufficient understanding of their purpose
- The prospects for getting these vaccines into resource-poor countries where the vaccine is least affordable; yet the need is greatest and the potential impact on women's health enormous.

These challenges need to be addressed, particularly the need to achieve primary prevention in countries with no means of secondary prevention. If that were to happen, HPV vaccination could rank alongside contraception as a means of preventing suffering and death in women worldwide.

Further reading

Brown D for the FUTURE Group (2007). HPV types 6, 11, 16, 18 vaccine: first analysis of cross protection against persistent infection, cervical intraepithelial neoplasia and adenocarcinoma *in-situ* caused by oncogenic types additional to 16/18. Presented at the 47th Annual Interscience Conference on Antimicrobial Agents and Chemotherapy (ICAAC), Chicago, 17–20 Sept. 2007.

Brown DR, Kjaer S, Sigurdsson K, Iversen O-E et al. (2009). The Impact of Quadrivalent Human Papillomavirus (HPV; Types 6, 11, 16, and 18) L1 Virus-Like Particle Vaccine on Infection and Disease Due to Oncogenic Nonvaccine HPV Types in Generally HPV-Naive Women Aged 16–26 Years. JID. **199**: 926–35.

FUTURE II Study Group (2007). Quadrivalent vaccine against human papilloma virus to prevent high-grade cervical lesions. *New England Journal of Medicine,* 356(19): 1915–27.

Garland SM, Hernandez-Avila M, Wheeler CM, *et al.* Females United to Unilaterally Reduce Endo/Ectocervical Disease (FUTURE) I Investigators. (2007). Quadrivalent vaccine against human papilloma virus to prevent anogenital diseases. *New England Journal od Medicine,* 356: 1928–43.

Harper DM, Franco EL, Wheeler C, *et al.* GlaxoSmithKline HPV Vaccine Study Group. (2004). Efficacy of a bivalent L1 virus-like particle vaccine in prevention of infection with human papilloma virus types 16 and 18 in young women: a randomised controlled trial. *Lancet,* 364: 1757–65.

Harper DM, Franco EL, Wheeler CM, *et al.* HPV Vaccine Study group. (2006). Sustained efficacy up to 4.5 years of a bivalent L1 virus-like particle vaccine against human papilloma virus types 16 and 18: follow-up from a randomised control trial. *Lancet,* 367: 1247–55.

Joura EA, Leodolter S, Hernandez-Avila M, *et al.* (2007). Efficacy of a quadrivalent prophylactic human papilloma virus (types 6, 11, 16, and 18) L1 virus-like-particle vaccine against high-grade vulval and vaginal lesions: a combined analysis of three randomised clinical trials. *Lancet,* 369: 1693–702.

Kitchener HC, Almonte M, Wheeler P, *et al.* ARTISTIC Trial Study Group. (2006). HPV testing in routine cervical screening: cross sectional data from the ARTISTIC trial. *British Journal of Cancer,* 95: 56–61.

Kjaer SK, van den Brule AJ, Paull G, *et al.* (2002). Type specific persistence of high risk human papilloma virus (HPV) as indicator of high grade cervical squamous intraepithelial lesions in young women: population based prospective follow up study. *British Medical Journal,* 325: 572.

Koutsky LA, Ault KA, Wheeler CM, *et al.* (2002). A controlled trial of a human papilloma virus type 16 vaccine. *New England Journal of Medicine,* 347: 1645–51.

Moscicki AB (2007). HPV infections in adolescents. *Disease Markers,* 23: 229–34.

Munoz N, Manalastas R Jr, Pitisuttihum P, Tresukosol D, Monsonego J *et al.* 2009. Safety, immunogenicity, and efficacy of quadrivalent human papillomavirus (types 6, 11, 16, 18) recombinant vaccine in women ages 24-45 years: a randomised, double-blind trial. *Lancet.* 373: 1949–57.

Paavonen J, Naud P, Salmeron J, Wheeler CM, Chow SN *et al.* (2009). Efficacy of human papillomavirus (HPV)-16/18 AS04-adjuvanted vaccine against cervical infection and precancer caused by oncogenic HPV types (PATRICIA): final analysis of a double-blind, randomised study in young women. *Lancet.* 374: 268–70.

Villa LL, Costa RL, Petta CA, *et al.* (2005). Prophylactic quadrivalent human papilloma virus (types 6, 11, 16, and 18) L1 virus-like particle vaccine in young women: a randomised double-blind placebo-controlled multicentre phase II efficacy trial. *Lancet Oncology,* 6: 271–8.

Chapter 9

Introduction of HPV prophylactic vaccination

Loretta Brabin

Key points

- Vaccine introduction requires complex decision making across a range of epidemiological, cost, social, and health system dimensions, and is a country-specific process.
- Countries currently introducing human papilloma virus (HPV) vaccination target different age groups and use various delivery models.
- HPV vaccine acceptance is expected to be high in Western countries, provided parents' concerns about safety and sexual risks are adequately addressed.
- Informed consent of adolescents should be a priority since vaccine acceptance is only the first step towards cervical cancer prevention.
- Delivery of HPV vaccines is feasible and could provide a platform for future adolescent vaccines and improved preventive care for this age group.

9.1 Health technological assessment

Gardasil® and Cervarix™ are approved vaccines for prevention of human papilloma virus (HPV) infection and cervical intraepithelial neoplasia (CIN), and their use should reduce cervical cancer. Although both vaccines have been licensed in countries all over the world, far fewer countries have proceeded to include HPV vaccination in their national immunization schedules. To promote evidence-based decision making, policy makers are advised to systematically address a series of complex issues, using a process commonly known as a Health Technology Assessment. Box 9.1 provides an outline of the main dimensions that are usually considered. Policy makers should review each dimension, taking into account the epidemiology of HPV infection and cervical cancer and how a vaccine will fit into existing health delivery systems. Economic analyses follow, to assess the

> **Box 9.1 Typical dimensions of a Health Technology Assessment**
> - Appraisal of infection/disease burden
> - Review of current preventive strategies
> - Mathematical models predicting vaccine impact
> - Cost-benefit and cost-effectiveness analyses
> - Evaluation of ethical, legal, and social issues
> - Study of organizational aspects and impact of vaccination on the health system.

potential cost-benefit and cost-effectiveness of HPV vaccination as many benefits occur in the medium to long term. Cost-effectiveness is generally a pre-requisite for government-funded vaccine programmes. Yet a level of uncertainty applies to the predictions generated by economic models as they are based on complex assumptions. Similarly, ethical, legal, and social issues should be evaluated, as well as the impact of vaccination on the organization of the health system (see Box 9.1.) This chapter will focus on the ethical, legal and social issues that arise in the course of vaccine implementation and will draw on examples of countries that have introduced HPV vaccination.

9.1.2 Determining the vaccine target group

Pre-adolescent girls are the primary target population for vaccination because immunization should ideally precede the onset of sexual activity. The vaccination of older adolescents is less cost-effective because sexual activity increases with age, and a proportion of girls will have acquired HPV 16/18 infections. Vaccination to induce herd immunity will not be easily achieved because some young women are currently and persistently infected, and males will continue to transmit HPV infection. Adolescent HPV sero-prevalence data provide a good indicator of HPV exposure and the optimum age to vaccinate. The UK recommendation to initiate vaccination in girls aged 12–13 was influenced by data showing that less than 5% of girls under the age of 14 were seropositive for any HPV type but after this age, sero-prevalence increased sharply. Alternatively, the optimum age for vaccination can be derived from the age distribution for reported onset of sexual intercourse.

Although age recommendations vary widely among countries that have introduced the vaccine, most authorities prioritise vaccination of young adolescents for routine vaccination. Countries recommending catch-up vaccination for older cohorts anticipate additional benefits due to protection against HPV types to which young women have not yet been exposed, as well as an earlier impact on HPV-related morbidity.

9.1.3 **Vaccine implementation**

A recent survey of 40 European countries indicated that 17 had made national recommendations for HPV vaccination that have, or will soon, be implemented. Most country recommendations were made before Cervarix was widely registered. Gardasil® has been approved for vaccine programmes in the United States, Canada, Australia, New Zealand, Spain, France, Switzerland and Sweden. The UK Health Authority, and more recently, The Netherlands, have chosen Cervarix™.

Since September 2008 girls aged 12 to 13 years in the UK are being immunised each year in a school-based programme as part of the routine National Health Service immunisation programme. In addition all girls aged 13 to 18 years are being offered the vaccine in a one-off "catch-up" programme. Provisional uptake figures for the first cohort of 12 to 13 year olds in Scotland, Wales and Northern Ireland have shown coverage levels exceeding 80% for the first and second doses overall. Scotland has also reported high uptake for older schoolgirls who have been vaccinated as part of the catch-up programme. No figures have yet been published for girls who have left school and were invited to attend community clinics and GP practices. In England just over one half of 16–18 year olds received their first vaccine dose. It is more difficult to achieve high coverage when the vaccine is offered by health providers outside the school setting to older girls who are making their own choices.

In many countries vaccination programmes are administered at the regional or provincial level and there are wide variations in who receives the vaccine and how it is delivered and reported. Australia has a school-based vaccination programme for females aged 12–18 years. Both New South Wales and Victoria vaccinated at least 70% of girls in most of the age cohorts. Interim data indicated that coverage for the third dose had fallen by about 10% across all territories. In Canada, all 10 provinces and the Yukon territory have completed their first year of a school-based programme. Acceptance rates ranged from 50–55% in Alberta and Manitoba to 83% in Newfoundland and Labrador. Acceptance was highest in Quebec, where 84% of nine-year olds and 87% of 14–15 year olds were vaccinated. In Alberta almost half of Catholic school boards barred in-school vaccination and although HPV vaccination was offered at public health clinics, compliance was low.

In much of Europe and the United States HPV vaccination is accessed "on demand" through a regular health provider or public health clinic. Even if supported by direct invitation and/or public education programmes, "on demand" programmes have a lower uptake and are more likely to miss lower socioeconomic groups and ethnic minorities. Only about one quarter of American 13–17 year olds have been vaccinated and some states will be introducing legislation for mandatory HPV vaccination before middle school entry to try and increase coverage.

Whatever the delivery strategy, implementation must be well planned and include easy access to the vaccine, clear vaccination protocols, health system linkages, well-trained providers, adequate insurance coverage, strong infrastructure for storage and dissemination of the vaccine, and quality control mechanisms.

9.1.4 Monitoring programme safety and effectiveness

Safety: Passive surveillance systems should be in place to monitor low incidence serious adverse events or unexpected vaccine side effects. In the United States monitoring is accomplished through the Vaccine Adverse Events Reporting System and the Center for Disease Control's Vaccine Safety Datalink. This includes surveillance of cohorts of recently vaccinated females and evaluation of outcomes of pregnancy among those pregnant at the time of delivery. In the UK adverse events are registered when individuals or health professionals complete a "yellow card" and send it to the Medicines and Healthcare Products Regulatory Agency. As of July 2009, 1913 reports had been registered, based on over one million administered vaccine doses. Most commonly reported reactions were nausea, headache and dizziness, but these did not occur at a higher frequency than described in the product information sheet. There were 281 cases that could not be classified as recognised Cervarix-associated side effects but none were attributed to the vaccine. In New South Wales, Australia, following the introduction of Gardasil® the anaphylaxis rate in the 2007 school-based programme was 2.6 per 100,000 doses (95% CI: 1.0 to 5.3 per 100,000 doses), which is higher than for other vaccines but still rare. One reason for this may be a high frequency of allergy-related conditions in young women. Both Cervarix™ and Gardasil® appear to be safe and well tolerated and most side effects disappear within the first day or two. Alarm stories that appear in the media after vaccine introduction have, nevertheless, the potential to lead to public demand for vaccine withdrawal.

Effectiveness: Systems may also need to be introduced to monitor vaccine effectiveness. The Australian Federal Government is establishing a HPV vaccine registry in order to:

- to provide details on participation rates;
- to record vaccine information that can be compared with cervical screening outcomes and cancer registries to assess the long-term effectiveness of HPV vaccination;
- to determine vaccination status or identify women who may require a booster dose;
- to collect statistics for general reporting;

- to inform participants about development within the HPV vaccination programme;
- to record details of vaccine providers;
- to allow a record to be anonymized if this is requested.

Consent is being obtained from parents for inclusion of a child's details on the National HPV Vaccination Program Register. The Register will receive data retrospectively from all states and territories and from all types of vaccination providers. Until the register is fully operational, no official statistics on coverage are available. In England, monthly provisional statistics are based on the school roll (for routine cohorts) or the population of Primary Care Trusts (for older catch-up cohorts). The official annual uptake is based on a more complex calculation but the monthly returns provide an ongoing monitoring tool. Primary Care Trusts return standardised survey forms using the Health Protection Informatics web-based reporting system. The Department of Health has also requested that the HPV immunisation records should be added to the future cervical screening records database. This is to improve evaluation of vaccine efficacy and to support health surveillance. It will also allow vaccinated women to follow a different recall system within the screening programme if future evidence supports this.

9.1.5 Funding adolescent vaccination

The cost of a vaccination programme includes provision of information and education, information technology systems, and staffing costs. Some of these are once-only costs, but routine delivery of a three-dose vaccine will necessarily compete for resources needed for other health targets, as both vaccines are expensive. It is estimated that in the United Kingdom, vaccination of adolescent girls under the National Health Service could add more than £72 million annually to the existing cervical cancer control programme, which already costs more than £150 million. In Europe only nine of 40 countries recently surveyed (Denmark, Germany, Greece, Italy, Luxembourg, Netherlands, Portugal, Spain and the UK) were offering HPV vaccination free of charge to at least one age-cohort of females, while an additional three countries (Belgium, France and Sweden) offer HPV vaccination on a co-payment system, ie. the national healthcare system reimburses only a percentage of the cost. In Switzerland HPV vaccination for primary and catch-up populations will be funded through mandatory health insurance. Austria will provide the vaccination free for 12 year olds but other populations will have to pay out-of-pocket.

In sum, vaccine policies balance political and economic realities with the scientific evidence base. Sometimes the introduction of new vaccines will be delayed or restricted because the cost to the health service, the insurance companies, or the tax payer, is too high. The risk is that recommending expensive vaccines without adequate public or social funding may lead to inequitable access and widen disparities in health between those who can afford private health care and those who cannot.

9.2 Ethical, legal and social challenges of adolescent HPV vaccination

9.2.1 Parental attitudes

Clinical and epidemiological aspects of a new technology are usually more thoroughly assessed than the ethical, legal, and social issues. Parental acceptability studies have recently increased as countries contemplate introducing an HPV vaccine. The majority indicate a high level of interest among parents, but low knowledge levels about HPV and cervical cancer. It has been concluded that wide-reaching public education about the benefits of the vaccine will be important to ensure a successful vaccination programme. Concerns were expressed that the knowledge that cervical cancer is caused by a sexually trans-mitted virus could stigmatize vaccination, as well as the disease, although mothers who had experienced the anxiety of an abnormal smear may be more sympathetic towards their daughter's vaccination. The other major issue was the perceived safety of the new vaccine which was prominent in most of the acceptability studies. A feasibility study (the Manchester study) that offered HPV vaccination to around 3000 12 year olds ahead of the UK national HPV programme reported that parents based their vaccine decision on information they had acquired from a variety of sources, principally from television, news-papers and the internet. HPV was not fundamentally questioned and the majority of parents were willing to accept a public health vaccine recommendation. Vaccine refusers were less reassured by the infor-mation provided and were more likely than acceptors to seek for additional information and to consult health professionals.

Some uncertainty among parents may still persist due to fears that vaccine acceptance conveys approval of adolescent sexual activity, concerns that vaccinated adolescents will take more sexual risks because they think they are protected, or because parents do not perceive their child to be at risk of a sexually transmitted infection. Some parents would prefer to have older children vaccinated, believing that HPV can, to some extent, be avoided or delayed by abstinence. There is no evidence to support the view that risk-taking behaviour would increase after vaccination, although no specific research re-lated to vaccination has been conducted. However, there is a wealth of research on adolescent behaviour, much of which leads to the conclusion that adolescent perception of risk is not the main driver of adolescent behaviour. The Manchester study reported that fewer that 5% of parents refused HPV vaccination on grounds that sexual risk-taking might increase.

9.2.2 Parental consent

The age of consent to medical procedures in many countries is 18 years although adolescents vaccinated at school generally require parental consent. In England laws have been enacted that permit a health provider to assess an individual child's understanding and competence to consent. Accordingly, consent for HPV vaccination is legally the child's. Although this is stated in the vaccine information sheet, parents are reassured that immunisation would be unlikely without their consent.

To vaccinate without parental consent might risk challenge by parents who consider it their right and responsibility to make health decisions on behalf of minors, especially for a vaccine against a sexually transmitted infection. In the United States, the attempt to make HPV vaccination a mandatory requirement for school entry has been opposed, even though parental opt-out rights would allow withdrawal on religious or secular grounds. One UK study also indicated that parents would be more likely to accept HPV vaccination if their consent was requested. Box 9.2. summarises the ethical perspectives of parents who either supported or opposed, adolescent vaccination without parental consent. Faced with an emotional response to any removal of the need for parental consent, policy makers may not be explicit about an adolescent's right to request the vaccine autonomously.

> **Box 9.2 Ethical views of parents who favour or oppose HPV vaccination without parental consent**
>
> Consent favoured
> For children
> - Who are well informed
> - Who are mature
> - Who need protection from naive or unrealistic parents.
>   Because it is inherently 'good' to prevent infection
> - Because children have a right to privacy
> - Because it is a child's right to decide.
>
> Consent opposed
> because
> - Parents should always be informed
> - Parents are responsible for a child's health
> - Children need to be guided by parents
> - Parents have a right to make decisions for their children
> - Sexual health clinics cause harm (oppose parental values).

In the Manchester study most parents said they discussed the vaccine decision with their daughters, but even so, about a third of parents who did not give consent stated that it was not the child's decision. School nurses were not pro-active in following up non-consented girls to determine their wishes. This could be attributed to confusion about laws and medical guidelines, the young age of girls, the desire to maintain good relationships with parents and schools and to some extent, the fact that many school nurses were parents themselves. Within the legal framework within which they operate, health providers have a duty of care to girls for whom no parental consent for HPV vaccination has been given. If the adolescent is marginal to the vaccine decision, she may be less motivated to positively engage in future preventive actions – notably cervical screening. Involving the adolescent, providing information at the time of vaccination and later in life, should be a priority of vaccine programmes.

9.2.3 Adolescent education and information

The quality of information given to adolescents is centrally important to cervical cancer prevention and this necessarily involves discussion of sexual issues. Some of this is basic biological and physiological information relating to the site and mode of infection and the link between HPV infection and cervical cancer (see Figure 9.1). They need also to understand that condoms may only partially protect them from HPV infection otherwise they may assume that vaccination is unnecessary if condoms are being used. Adolescents may have difficulty understanding the mechanism of action of HPV vaccines or be concerned that vaccination could cause HPV infection.

The following have been recommended as important concepts to consider when designing HPV educational strategies:

- They must be tailored to the specific source of information (eg educational videos, on-line materials, school-based sexuality education etc);
- Their design should take account of adolescent cognitive development, given that this is a complex topic;
- The sexually transmitted nature of the infection could cause anxiety or ambiguity;
- Key messages should be defined. These should include the mechanism of action of HPV vaccines, possible side effects, the importance of adhering to the vaccine schedule and the fact that the vaccine only protects against specific HPV types.

Information on cervical cancer prevention will need to be reinforced because of the long gap between vaccination and entry to the cervical screening programme (at least in England, where screening starts after the 25th birthday).

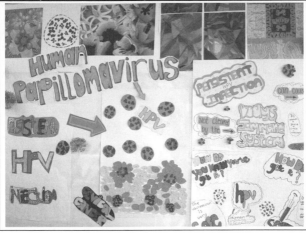

Figure 9.1 Art work produced by school children learning about prevention of cervical cancer. Image reproduced courtesy of Lorraine A Vallely

9.3 **Ongoing issues**

9.3.1 **The challenge of a three-dose vaccine**

The challenges of incorporating a three-dose vaccine schedule into busy secondary schools cannot be under-estimated. The Department of Health in the UK has departed from the vaccine manufacturer's recommended dosing schedule of 0,1 and 6 months to allow delivery of Dose 2 between four and eight weeks, and Dose 3 up to 12 months after Dose 1. This is to facilitate follow up of girls who missed their third dose when the vaccine teams return to start vaccinating a new cohort of girls one year later. This policy prioritises completion of the three doses over maintenance of the dosing schedule. In Canada, British Columbia, Quebec and Nova Scotia are conducting a clinical trial to study the safety and effectiveness of giving younger girls two doses instead of the current three-dose regimen. No results have been published so far. In Quebec, girls participating in the immunisation programme were given the first two doses of the vaccine in Grade 4, but the third dose will only be given in Grade 9. There is no immunogenicity or efficacy data available to justify this approach at the present time.

9.3.2 **Vaccinating boys**

All national vaccine programmes have limited their target population to adolescent girls. Since the purpose of HPV vaccination is prevention of cervical disease, vaccinating girls alone is sufficient to achieve a linear reduction in prevalence amongst girls. One of the problems of a sex-specific vaccine is that males may remain ignorant about their role in transmitting the virus. Without some understanding of HPV and cervical cancer, men might perceive themselves to be less at risk of contracting a sexually transmitted infection from women and take fewer risk-reducing precautions. One recent study reported that men are moderately interested in HPV vaccination to prevent genital warts and male cancers, but less interested in vaccination as a means to protect their partners from cervical cancer. Mathematical modelling studies have suggested that increasing coverage of women is always more cost effective than introducing men to the vaccination programme.

9.3.3 Building the prevention platform

Apart from boosters to increase or maintain effective protection derived from childhood vaccination, there is an expanding platform of newly recommended adolescent vaccinations. In addition to hepatitis B, some countries recommend meningococcal conjugate, as well as the tetanus-diphtheria-acellular pertussis vaccines.

There is a raft of vaccines under development that could target adolescents, such as herpes simplex virus-2. Adherence to the recommended HPV schedule provides an opportunity to introduce infrastructural changes in adolescent care that could enhance the scope of preventive care for this age group.

Further reading

Boot HJ, Wallenburg I, De Melker HE, Mangen M-J M, Gerritsen AAM, Van der Maas NA, Berkhof J, Meijer CJLM, Kimman TG (2007). Assessing the introduction of universal human papillomavirus vaccination for preadolescent girls in The Netherlands. *Vaccine*, **25**: 6245–6256.

Brabin L, Roberts SA, Stretch R, Baxter D, Chambers G, Kitchener H, McCann R (2008). Uptake of first two doses of human papillomavirus vaccine by adolescent school girls in Manchester: prospective cohort study. *BMJ*, **16**: 53–58.

Brabin L. Roberts SA, Kitchener HC (2007). A semi-qualitative study of attitudes to vaccinating adolescents against human papillomavirus without parental consent. *BMC Public Health*, **7**: 20.

Brotherton JML, Deeks SL, Campbell-Lloyd S, Misrachi A, Passaris I, Peterson K, Pitcher H, Scully M, Watson W, Webby R (2008). Interim estimates of human papillomavirus vaccination coverage in the school-based program in Australia. *CDI*, **32**: 457–461

Colucci R, Hryniuk W, Savage C (2008). HPV vaccination programs in Canada. Are we hitting the mark? Report Card on Cancer in Canada: 7–10.

European Cervical Cancer Association (2009). HPV vaccination across Europe. Available at: http://www.ecca.info/fileadmin/user_upload/HPV_Vaccination/ECCA_HPV_Vaccination_April_2009.pdf

Gerend MA and Barley J (2009). Human papillomavirus vaccine acceptability among young adult men. *Sex Transm Dis*, **36**:58–62.

Jit M, Vyse A, Borrow R, Pebody R, Soldan K, Miller E (2007). Prevalence of human papillomavirus antibodies in young female subjects in England. *Br J Cancer*, **97**: 989–991.

Kollar LM and Kahn JA (2008). Education about human papillomavirus and human papillomavirus vaccines in adolescents. *Curr Opin Obstet Gynecol*, **20**: 479–483.

Koulova A, Tsui J, Irwin K, Van Damme P, Biellik R, Aguado MT (2008). Country recommendations on the inclusion of HPV vaccines in national immunization programmes among high-income countries, June 2006–January 2008. *Vaccine*, **26**: 6529–6541.

Raffle AE (2007). Challenges of implementing human papillomavirus (HPV) vaccination policy. *BMJ*, **335**: 375–377.

Stretch R, McCann R, Roberts SA, Elton P. Baxter D, Brabin L. A qualitative study to assess school nurses' views on vaccinating 12-13 year old school girls against human papillomavirus without parental consent. *BMC Public Health 2009*: **9**:254.

Part 4

Challenges and future developments

Chapter 10

HPV vaccination in the developing world

Rengaswamy Sankaranarayanan
and Catherine Sauvaget

Key points

- Four-fifths of the cervical cancer burden is in the developing world where there is a lack of effective screening.
- The potential to reduce cervical cancer by human papilloma virus (HPV) vaccination in developing countries is challenged by cost and lack of effective vaccine delivery platforms for children and adolescents.
- Other challenges include the following:
- Sensitivies of using a vaccine preventing an STI in girls
- Lack of awareness, public demand, and political will
- Lack of coordination between cancer control, sexual/reproductive health, and vaccine delivery services.
- Local production of vaccines at reduced cost, logistically feasible efficacious vaccine regimes, and strengthening vaccine delivery infrastructure for children and adolescents will be required for successful HPV vaccination in developing countries.

10.1 Burden of cervical cancer in developing countries

Cervical cancer is a global public health problem that disproportionately affects poor women in developing countries in sub-Saharan Africa, Central and South America, and South and South-East Asia (Figure 10.1; see also Chapter 4). There is a more than 20-fold difference between the highest and the lowest incidence rates of cervical cancer worldwide. In many developing countries, age-standardized incidence and mortality rates of cervix cancer exceed 30 and 12 per 100 000 women, respectively, as opposed to much lower rates in developed countries (Figure 10.1). Of the estimated

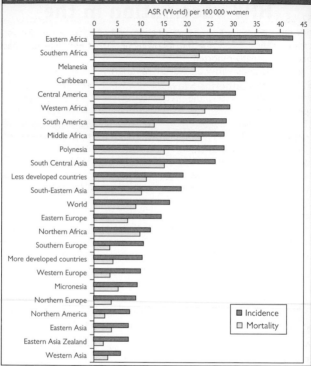

Figure 10.1 Cervical cancer incidence and mortality rate in selected regions (see Ferlay 2002). Figure created by Dr Sankar, GLOBOCAN 2002 (mortality statistics)

5.1 million new cancer cases and 2.9 million cancer deaths in women in the world around 2002, cervical cancer accounted for 493 000 cases and 273 000 deaths. Over 80% of this burden is experienced in developing countries, where women at the highest risk of death from it have the least access to screening, early diagnosis, and treatment. While widespread Pap smear screening has contributed to a substantial decline in cervical cancer mortality in developed countries over the last five decades, cervical cancer still remains the largest single cause of years of life lost (YLL) to cancer in the developing world, with devastating effects on the well-being of families and society at large. With this background of lack of screening programmes in many developing countries, the prospect for human papilloma virus (HPV) vaccination to control cervical cancer is discussed briefly in this chapter.

10.2 **HPV infection and cervical cancer**

The fact that cervical neoplasia is caused by persistent infection with one or more of the 15 high-risk HPVs (16, 18, 31, 33, 35, 39, 45, 51, 52, 56, 58, 59, 68, 73, and 82) has provided an exciting opportunity to prevent cervical cancer by vaccination. Very high relative risk for cervical cancer exceeding 100, following persistent HPV infection, has been consistently reported.

In a meta-analysis involving 14 595 cases of invasive cervical cancer, 87% contained one or more of the oncogenic HPV genotypes that cause cervical cancer; the frequency of HPV in cervical cancer specimens ranged from 86% to 94% by different regions of the world (Table 10.1) (see Smith 2007). HPV 16 was the most common (ranging from 52% in Asia to 58% in Europe) and HPV 18 the second most common (ranging from 13% in South/Central America to 22% in North America) found in cervical cancer specimens. Overall HPV 16/18 frequency in cervical cancer specimens was 70% (Figure 10.2), and varied from 65% in South/Central America to 76% in North America (Table 10.1). HPV 31, 33, 35, 45, 52, and 58 are the six next most important types. Overall, HPV prevalence in 7084 high-grade cervical intraepithelial neoplasia (CIN2 and 3) specimens was 85%, ranging from 78% in Asia to 88% in Europe (Table 10.1) and the combined HPV 16 and 18 prevalence was 52% (Figure 10.2).

10.3 **Challenges for HPV vaccination in national immunization programmes in developing countries**

While HPV vaccination provides an important emerging avenue for cervical cancer prevention, and currently available evidence supports the introduction of HPV vaccines, there are several challenges and uncertainties that need to be resolved before HPV vaccination can be widely implemented through public health services in high-risk developing countries. These include affordability because of current high costs of the available vaccines, feasibility, acceptability, and logistics of vaccine delivery, such as the need for three doses spread over 6 months, and improved strategies and vaccine platforms to reach out to pre- or early-adolescent girls. In addition, there are uncertainties regarding long-term immunogenicity and efficacy in preventing cervical neoplasia, cross-protection against HPV infections not targeted by the vaccine antigens and the efficacy of different, more logistically feasible dose regimes in inducing and maintaining immunogenicity and long-term protection against cervical neoplasia.

Table 10.1 **Prevalence of human papilloma virus (HPV) type 16/18 among women with invasive cervical cancer and with high-grade cervical intraepilitheal lesions (see Smith 2007)**

Regions	HPV prevalence (% of all cases tested)							
	Invasive cervical cancer (14 595 cases)				Cervical intraepithelial neoplasia grade 2 and 3 lesions (7094 cases)			
	Any HPV	HPV 16	HPV 18	HPV 31, 33, 35, 45, 52, 58	Any HPV	HPV 16	HPV 18	HPV 31, 33, 35, 45, 52, 58
Africa	93.9	54.5	15.5	22.3	85.2	40.9	7.4	34.9
Asia	85.9	52.0	14.9	19.8	78.0	33.7	6.6	37.2
Europe	85.7	58.1	15.7	14.7	87.8	51.5	6.0	30.5
North America	86.9	54.2	22.2	13.0	85.6	45.3	9.8	36.1
South/Central America	91.1	52.4	12.7	25.5	84.4	40.5	7.5	33.7
Oceania	88.7	56.5	21.1	10.6	95.8	33.3	10.4	31.3
Total	87.3	54.4	15.9	19.1	84.9	45.4	6.9	34.1

Source: Adapted from Smith, Clifford, and the WHO report by Sankaranarayanan.

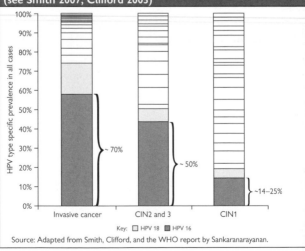

Figure 10.2 **HPV type specific prevalence in cervical neoplasia (see Smith 2007; Clifford 2005)**

Key: ☐ HPV 18   ■ HPV 16

Source: Adapted from Smith, Clifford, and the WHO report by Sankaranarayanan.

These aspects need to be resolved to achieve adequate support for a global policy recommendation for the introduction of HPV vaccine to gain momentum.

As mentioned in Chapters 8, 12, and 14, data pertaining to long-term immunogenicity, efficacy in preventing cervical cancer, the need for booster doses, cross-protection, and developments such as newer generations of vaccines, including high-risk types other than HPV 16/18, will take several years to emerge. This will limit to a certain extent the application of HPV vaccination throughout the world. Similarly, sociocultural factors will affect the acceptability of the HPV vaccine globally, but challenges related to the affordability and acceptability of the vaccine, introduction of new vaccines, and vaccine delivery are highly relevant to the introduction of these vaccines in national immunization programs in poor countries.

10.4 Challenges in introducing a new vaccine in developing countries

Immunization delivery for infants is the most successful public health initiative in the world, and the infrastructure of trained staff, cold chain and logistics, clinics and outreach services, and information systems is a resource that may be potentially used to deliver new vaccines. Factors such as political awareness, will, public demand, availability of resources, donor pressure, and competing priorities are major determinants for the successful introduction of any new vaccine in developing countries. Developing countries have few resources to devote to introducing new vaccines and several new vaccines against major killers of children such as pneumococcal pneumonia, rotavirus vaccine, Japanese encephalitis, and meningococcal meningitis will compete for these limited resources. The impact of these vaccines against infections that kill children will be seen long before that of HPV vaccine. Rational decision-making to select new vaccines (e.g. HPV vaccine) among these potentially competing priorities are further complicated by the difficulties in engaging the immunization (traditionally paediatric) community and the reproductive health/ gynaecology and cancer control communities in a coordinated fashion.

In developing countries, expensive and new vaccines are often available only in the private sector, that is, for the better-off, and the rest of the general public have to wait for decades before it becomes available in their health services. For example, it took more than two decades for hepatitis B vaccine (HBV) to become available in medium-resourced countries after the licensing of the vaccine in developed countries. Most developing countries are yet to introduce Haemophilus influenzae b (Hib) vaccine, although it has been in use in developed countries for more than two decades. The availability of newer vaccines on the private market may contribute, to a certain extent, to an eventual wider availability and demand for introduction in the public sector in the long run, as it may prove educative for physicians, decision makers, and the public.

10.5 **Vaccine costs and affordability**

A single dose of a 3 dose HPV vaccine schedule currently costs over US$120 in different developed and developing countries. The current extremely high costs of the vaccine, made in industrialized countries, make them unaffordable for either public health use or use by the low- and medium-socio-economic groups in many developing countries. The high cost is the major barrier for the rapid introduction and widespread use of HPV vaccine in immunization programmes in poor countries. It is impossible for the public health sector to consider implementing HPV vaccine at these costs, given the fact that the entire vaccine antigens used for infant vaccination in different developing countries cost less than US$5 per child. The affordability of these infant vaccines is due to the production of these antigens in developing countries such as India, China, Indonesia, South Korea, South Africa, and Brazil among others. Unless the HPV vaccine costs dramatically less than current prices, and until it falls at least to the level of HBV vaccines, it is not possible for the public health sector in almost all sub-Saharan African countries, and most Asian and Latin American countries to afford this vaccine. Local production options in developing countries leading to reduced prices and cheaper alternative technologies for HPV vaccine production will prove critical for their rapid introduction in poor countries.

10.6 **Strategies and infrastructure for vaccine procurement and delivery**

Policies and strategies for the national immunization programmes in developing countries are determined nationally, although they are heavily influenced by policies of the World Health Organisation (WHO), Expanded Programme on Immunization (EPI), and donor organizations. Vaccines targeting children are predominantly delivered in public health services through a national immunization program (NIP) formulated and supported by national governments, with or without additional financial and technical support from selected donor countries and organizations. The EPI began in 1974 with six antigens, but now includes at least eight in its globally recommended schedule; Bacillus Calmette-Guérin (BCG) against tuberculosis, oral polio vaccine, diphtheria–tetanus–pertussis (DTP), hepatitis B vaccine (HBV), and measles-containing vaccines in the infant immunization schedule, and tetanus–toxoid (TT)-containing vaccines for women of childbearing age. The coverage for EPI vaccines varies considerably among developing countries (Table 10.2).

Current vaccine delivery strategies include activities such as immunization, growth monitoring and nutrition, family planning, antenatal care, basic treatment of common childhood illnesses, and so on, at fixed sites in primary health care services such as health centres, and through mass campaigns, for example, pulse polio programmes. In addition, vaccines are purchased and prescribed to individuals through the private sector, and individuals or private insurance schemes pay for these services. Delivery of booster doses following primary immunization in infancy and the introduction of new vaccines in most developing countries are heavily influenced by the level of economic development, of health service infrastructure, financial resources, the relative priority, and the epidemiological patterns of disease and political considerations. For example, a vast majority of African countries and many South and East Asian countries, and some Latin American countries lack a policy for administration of booster doses in pre-school children and vaccination to persons aged 9–20 in their routine national immunization schedule.

Coverage for vaccination of school children varies widely across the world. HPV vaccination currently targets pre-adolescent and adolescent girls because the vaccine is highly immunogenic at that age and the risk of having acquired a high-risk HPV infection is low. Integration of HPV vaccines into existing vaccine platforms could prove challenging in resource-poor settings since a comprehensive vaccination delivery infrastructure for adolescent vaccines is poorly developed or almost absent in most of these countries and, in many settings, new systems will be needed to reach young adolescents. The logistics of supplies of sterile syringes and needles, supplies for infection prevention, storage and transport of vaccines, and of teams in the context of an adolescent vaccination programme may also prove complex.

Another challenge is to find a conduit to ensure youth accessibility. In developing countries, schools are often used as a focus for adolescent vaccination. This can be problematic because school attendance during later adolescence may be low; girls may be less likely to be in school than boys and often leave school early. Therefore, the poor who need the vaccine most are most likely not to be in school in many of the poorer countries. In India, it is reported that less than 50% of school-aged girls attend school in some states. In areas where the rate of school enrolment among girls is low, community-based efforts to reach girls outside school need to be explored.

Table 10.2 Target infant populations (%) vaccinated by EPI vaccine antigens in selected developing countries: WHO–UNICEF estimates for 2005

Vaccine	India (620 US$)	Bangladesh (440 US$)	Phillippines (1170 US$)	Nigeria (430 $)	Senegal (630 US$)	Angola (930 US$)	Argentina (3580 US$)	Brazil (3000 US$)	Mexico (6790 US$)
BCG	75	99	91	48	92	61	99	99	99
DPT3	59	88	79	25	84	47	92	96	98
Polio3	58	88	80	39	84	46	92	98	98
MCV	58	81	80	35	74	45	99	99	96
Hib3	–	–	–	–	18	–	92	96	98
Hepatitis B	8	62	44	–	84	–	87	92	98

* US Dollars per capita gross national income (GNI); DPT3: 3 doses of triple vaccine; Polio3:3 doses of oral polio vaccine; MCV: measles containing vaccine; Hib3: 3 doses of Haemophilus influenzae type b vaccine (see http://www.who.int). Adapted from Smith, Clifford, and the WHO report by Sankararanayanan.

10.7 **Frequency of vaccination and revaccination**

In countries with limited resources and health care infrastructure, coverage for re-vaccination/booster is often lower than those requiring a single shot of the vaccine. For instance, the coverage for the first dose of polio vaccine or triple vaccine is substantially higher than that for three doses in many developing countries. Thus, the current regime of three doses of HPV vaccine over 6 months for those aged over 9 makes it difficult to achieve high coverage. It is not known yet if fewer than three doses can provide adequate long-term protection against infection and CIN, and this needs to be addressed to ascertain whether vaccination delivery costs could be reduced and coverage improved.

10.8 **Sociocultural challenges**

Parental consent is a critical factor in HPV vaccine acceptability. Parental beliefs, such as that a vaccine against a sexually transmitted infection (STI) will encourage children to become sexually promiscuous and that children will not have sex before marriage, and therefore do not need the vaccine, exist and may interfere with vaccine coverage. Vaccine associated with an STI may generate rumours that vaccination is a plot to sterilize girls and young women. This misunderstanding may be further potentiated in environments characterized by mistrust of governmental health care initiatives, particularly in developing countries. The general lack of awareness about the relationship between HPV infection and cervical cancer may further complicate the scenario. Lack of demand for HPV vaccine, sociocultural sensitivities regarding HPV infection, and the promotion of HPV vaccine may lead to inadequate political will and lack of public support. For better acceptance, HPV vaccine should be promoted as a cervical cancer prevention vaccine rather than a vaccine for prevention of a sexually transmitted viral infection. If it is promoted as a vaccine for the prevention of an STI, considerable controversies which centre on moral issues may decrease vaccine acceptability. This may not be a major problem in countries where contraceptive practices, including emergency contraception, are widely practised and accessible. The HIV/AIDS community has great experience in dealing with cultural issues involving sexuality, and will be very helpful in designing materials and training health care workers to discuss these issues on a country-specific basis.

10.9 **Prospects for HPV vaccine in developing countries**

Much effort, political will, and money will be needed to avoid the tragedy of delaying the benefits of HPV vaccine to women in the developing world. In order to save women's lives, developing countries should urgently explore local production options, price negotiation, and secure financing. The affordability of vaccines and future evidence base for the still unanswered questions related to long-term immunogenicity, cross-protection, alternate dose regimes, and ultimate reduction in the burden of disease following immunization are critical for the introduction of HPV vaccines in poor countries. Coordinated investments in health service platforms that support other interventions such as nutritional supplements, health promotion, and provision of sex education for adolescents and repro-ductive health information, will help in organizing and strengthening adolescent and pre-adolescent vaccine platforms, setting the stage for potential future addition of HPV vaccines, and possible new vaccines against HIV infection or tuberculosis.

Further reading

Agosti JM, and Goldie SJ (2007). Introducing HPV vaccine in developing countries–key challenges and issues. *New England Journal of Medicine*, **56**: 1908–10.

Clifford G, Rana RK, Franceschi S, Smith J, Gough G, Pimenta JM (2005). Human papilloma virus genotype distribution in low-grade cervical lesions: comparison by geographic region and with cervical cancer. *Cancer Epidemiological Biomarker*, **14**: 1157–64.

Ferlay J, Bray F, Pisani P, Parkin DM (2004). *Cancer incidence, mortality and prevalence worldwide. GLOBOCAN 2002*. IARC Cancer Base 5(version 2.0). IARC Press, Lyon.

FUTURE II Study Group. (2007). Quadrivalent vaccine against human papilloma virus to prevent high-grade cervical lesions. *New England Journal of Medicine*, **356**: 1915–27.

Http://www.who.int/vaccines-documents/GlobalSummary/GlobalSummary.pdf

Jacob M, Bradley J, Barone MA (2005). Human papilloma virus vaccines: what does the future hold for preventing cervical cancer in resource-poor settings through immunization programs? *Sexually Transmitted Diseases*, **32**: 635–40.

Kane MA, Sherris J, Coursaget P, Aguado T, Cutts F (2006). Chapter 15: HPV vaccine use in the developing world. *Vaccine*, **24**(Suppl 3): S132.

Koutsky LA and Harper DM (2006) Chapter 13. Current findings from prophylactic HPV vaccine trials. *Vaccine*, **24**(Suppl 3): S114.

Muñoz N, Bosch FX, de Sanjosé S, Herrero R, Castellsagué X, Shah KV, et al. (2003). Epidemiologic classification of human papilloma virus types associated with cervical cancer. *New England Journal of Medicine*, **348**: 518–27.

Sankaranarayanan R, Budukh AM, Rajkumar R (2001). Effective screening programmes for cervical cancer in low- and middle-income developing countries. *Bulletin of the World Health Organisation*, **79**: 954–62.

Smith J, Lindsay L, Hoots B, Keys J, Franceschi S, Winer R, et al. (2007). Human papilloma virus type distribution in invasive cervical cancer and high-grade cervical lesions: a meta-analysis update. *International Journal of Cancer*, **121**: 621–32.

Chapter 11

Screening post vaccination

Patrick Walker, Adeola Atilade,
and Henry C Kitchener

Key points

- The current NHS CSP is successful in avoiding 75% of cervical cancers that would otherwise occur.
- The current cervical screening programme will remain the major means of cervical cancer protection for the screened population for at least 10 years, by which time the vaccinated generation will have reached the threshold age for cervical screening.
- Modifications to the current screening programme will take account of the vaccination programme that is to be introduced, as well as emerging evidence regarding the impact of vaccination on cervical disease.
- Challenges during the transition from an unvaccinated to a vaccinated population should include maintaining awareness of the continuing need for cervical screening.
- It is likely that after vaccination there will be greater reliance on human papilloma virus (HPV) testing as the primary screening test, which will present challenges in maintaining skills in cytology screening.

11.1 The current screening programme

11.1.1 The call and recall programme

As described in Chapter 1, the English NHS CSP provides a call and recall programme for women invited for cervical cytology screening, starting at age 25, continuing every 3 years until age 50 and subsequently every 5 years until age 65. In Scotland, Wales, and Northern Ireland screening starts at 20 years. Between 1988 and 2004, the UK-wide programme resulted in a 7% year-on-year reduction in the incidence of cervical cancer such that the number of cervical cancer deaths has almost halved since 1988, with fewer than 1000 per year in England. It is estimated that approximately 70% of cases that would otherwise occur are prevented by the screening programme. The principal reasons for the success of the programme have been high coverage of the population and rigorous quality assurance across the entire programme from smear taking to colposcopy. The recent change to a start age of 25 years from age 20 has been controversial but was introduced in England because there was a risk that over-treatment could do more harm than any impact of cervical cancer, which is very rare between 20 and 24 years.

The title of this chapter suggests that primary prevention by vaccination will affect the susceptibility of the population to cervical cancer, which will require adjustment to cervical screening. There has been a lot of discussion regarding the case for human papilloma virus (HPV) testing instead of cytology as the primary test to achieve greater sensitivity. Prophylactic vaccination against HPV provides an added rationale to use an HPV test as the 'gatekeeper' for the necessity of further screening as a means of secondary prevention.

Although the sensitivity of high-risk (HR) HPV testing is higher than that of cervical cytology, it is less specific; indeed, the prevalence of positive HPV testing in the under 30-year age group can reach 20%, leading some to suggest that HPV screening should not be used in women under the age of 30–35. Using reflex cytology to triage would still select about 10% who would be HPV positive/cytology negative. So, if we are to use HPV testing we need to understand the risks of being HPV positive with negative cytology. There may be a role for HPV typing, as we know that HPV 16 carries the greatest risk.

HPV testing is being gradually implemented as a triage for women with low-grade cervical cytological abnormalities, that is, borderline change and mild dyskaryosis, to identify those women who are at risk of high-grade CIN and who can then be referred for colposcopy. Using HPV testing as a test of cure following treatment for CIN, either alone or in combination with a cytology test, will allow an earlier return to standard recall for HPV negative women.

11.1.2 **The continuance of the current programme**

Notwithstanding the establishment of a vaccination programme in current teenagers, there will be a need for cervical screening to continue. There are several reasons to justify this. First, although the clinical trials have suggested that efficacy for the primary composite endpoint of protection against HPV 16 and HPV 18 associated high-grade disease and cancer is over 90%, follow-up has only reached 5 years and there are, as yet, insufficient data to confirm that this protection will be maintained. Second, the protection against HPV 16 and HPV 18 high-grade disease and cancer in the intention to treat population was only 44% and therefore, although vaccinated, many of these women will remain at risk for the development of disease and will require regular screening. Furthermore, the relative efficacy of the vaccine against all high-risk HPV type associated CIN2, CIN3, CGIN, and cancer in the intention to treat analysis of the whole trial population was less than 20%. It is therefore essential that vaccinated women are offered cervical screening.

Irrespective of HPV vaccination the results of several randomized trials are becoming available and support is growing for HPV as a primary test to increase sensitivity, with reflex cytology for HPV-positive women. The advent of HPV vaccination is strengthening the case for HPV-based screening because fewer women will be HR HPV positive, and therefore, fewer women will need cytology. HR HPV-negative women are considered to be at very low risk of CIN3, and therefore, not requiring cytology. Furthermore, the protective effect of HPV testing may well extend beyond 3 years, allowing consideration of extending the screening interval.

11.2 **Challenges during the transition**

Cervical cytology screening is a skilled and repetitive task. The intro-duction of liquid-based cytology (LBC), which has reduced the unsat-isfactory smear rate, has been well received by cytoscreeners. As the impact of the introduction of vaccination is felt, there will be a reduction of up to 50% of high-grade cytology abnormalities, but much less of an impact on low-grade abnormalities. At present, about 10% of screened slides contain some abnormality and about 1.5% show high-grade change. This will sometimes be seen in only a few cells on the slide. The reduction in the prevalence of abnormalities in the screened smears may reduce the positive predictive value (PPV) of the test because the threshold for calling high grade may fall. There is also the potential for overcall of trivial abnormalities by those anxious not to miss the very occasional abnormal cell.

The prospect that the pre-eminence of cervical cytology will diminish in the years ahead could aggravate staff shortages and difficulties in recruitment and retention of staff, if the perception is that there will be a massive reduction in cytology screening. There would be problems associated with increased labour costs per individual employed, difficul-ties with quality assurance, and challenges to training programmes.

As far as colposcopy is concerned, there is increasing evidence to suggest that its diagnostic accuracy is not much greater than cytology. It remains the key tool to determine the site of disease, where to biopsy, which lesions require treatment and which do not, which require conization, and which harbour a significant risk of cancer and which do not. Colposcopy also allows the tailoring of treatment for each woman to effect adequate excision while minimizing damage to normal tissues. The introduction of the formal BSCCP/RCOG training programme and re-certification maintains the high standard of colposcopy in the United Kingdom, but a diminishing referral rate, with a lower prevalence of significant disease, will have the same implications for training and quality assurance as for cytoscreeners. Fewer colposcopists will be required if sufficient case-load to maintain skills is to be a quality standard.

11.3 Developments in screening post vaccination

The potential to introduce HPV testing to the current NHSCSP already exists and will almost certainly occur for triage for low-grade cytology changes and post-treatment 'test of cure' before the effect of vaccination is realized. There is already evidence to support primary screening with HPV testing to increase sensitivity, particularly for the over 30-year-old group. Because the purpose of primary prevention is to render women negative for HPV 16 and 18 (and perhaps in the future, a wider range of types), it seems logical to screen initially for HPV. If HPV negative, that woman can be considered free of risk as far as cervical cancer is concerned for 3–5 years, according to the woman's age. Women at risk by virtue of testing positive for HPV could have reflex cytology. Those with abnormal cytology could be referred for colposcopy; those with negative cytology would require follow-up in 3 years though HPV typing may have a role in stratifying risk. The use of HPV as a first screen would reduce the need for cytology to around 15–20% of what is currently undertaken. Decisions as to the latter will be based on the results from pivotal European randomized trials of HPV testing, and crucially cost-effectiveness.

One interesting concept for HPV testing is self-testing for 'hard to reach' women. The approach has been shown to be feasible with only a small drop in sensitivity. Advances in our understanding of cell biology will lead to more sophisticated biomarkers, both of HPV infection and of perturbed cellular growth. The major problem with HPV screening is the lack of test specificity, and so HPV tests based on HR-HPV RNA and biomarkers both dependent and independent of HPV, for example, p16^{ink} and MCM, respectively, could be helpful in triaging positive HPV results.

All women, whether vaccinated or not, will need to be offered screening in the foreseeable future. Those women who have been vaccinated will be at reduced risk of developing cancer, although the risk of acquiring a non-16, non-18 oncogenic HPV type will not be affected unless cross-protection can be demonstrated. Current trials of HPV screening may well provide strong evidence for HPV screening, with scope for increased screening intervals; however strategies

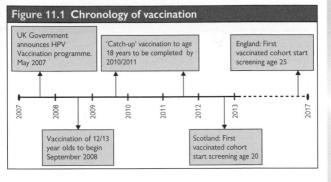

Figure 11.1 Chronology of vaccination

for HPV-positive tests, especially in young women, would need to be developed. The challenge of adapting cervical screening accounting vaccination will need to be addressed prior to the onset of screening of the vaccinees (2012 in Scotland, Jan 2017 in England) (Figure 11.1).

11.4 Chronology of vaccination

It has been suggested that HPV testing should be used in women over 30 years, but the screening programme should be kept as simple as possible, avoiding different categories of tests for different women. This in itself will be challenging but the real goal should be to 'de-intensify' secondary screening because of reduced risk overall, thus rendering vaccination more cost-effective. A number of individuals have expressed disagreement with the increased age to commence screening, though 25 years has now been recommended by the International Agency for Research on Cancer (IARC). The argument put forth by some is that earlier sexual debut will result in earlier development of CIN3, and in a few, cancer. Moreover, concern has been expressed that non-uptake of screening at 25 years (and uptake in the 25–30 age group has fallen) could result in increased rates of cancer. HPV vaccination will reduce the risk to the population with the likelihood of early cancer becoming far less; thus there will be a reduced rationale for any reconsideration of 20 years as the onset of screening. The devolved governments of Scotland, Wales and Northern Ireland which have retained 20 years to begin screening, may reconsider following the adoption of vaccination.

A proposal for how cervical screening may evolve is shown in Figure 11.2.

121

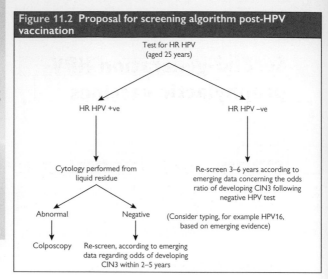

Figure 11.2 Proposal for screening algorithm post-HPV vaccination

Test for HR HPV
(aged 25 years)

HR HPV +ve

HR HPV −ve

Cytology performed from
liquid residue

Re-screen 3–6 years according to
emerging data concerning the odds
ratio of developing CIN3 following
negative HPV test

(Consider typing, for example HPV16,
based on emerging evidence)

Abnormal

Negative

Colposcopy

Re-screen, according to emerging
data regarding odds of developing
CIN3 within 2–5 years

Chapter 12

Second-generation HPV prophylactic vaccines

Richard BS Roden

Key points

- The approved HPV vaccines, Gardasil® and Cervarix®, prevent infection by a subset of oncogenic HPV types, necessitating the development of highly multivalent L1 VLP vaccines or developing L2 as a single broadly protective antigen.
- Vaccine may be too expensive for use in developing countries where >80% of cervical cancer cases occur.
- Potential second-generation HPV preventive vaccines nearing clinical study include the following:
  - L1 expressed in *Salmonella typhi* for low-cost manufacture and oral delivery.
  - L1 capsomeres purified from *Escherichia coli* for low-cost manufacture and greater temperature stability.
  - L2 protein purified from *E. coli* for low-cost manufacture and broad protection.
- A combination of tiered pricing, local manufacture, and new technology is required to realize the full potential of HPV vaccination worldwide.

12.1 The need for second-generation HPV preventive vaccines

Human papilloma viruses (HPVs) are small, non-enveloped DNA viruses that induce epithelial tumors (warts) of skin or mucosa. The majority of HPV infections produce benign tumors with limited growth that often spontaneously regress. Of the nearly 200 genotypes of HPV that have been identified, approximately 15 have been classified as oncogenic: HPV 16 and HPV 18 are the most common types detected in cervical cancer, whereas types HPV 31, HPV 33, HPV 35, HPV 45, HPV 51, HPV 52, HPV 56, HPV 58, etc., are found less frequently. Persistent oncogenic HPV infection is a necessary but not sufficient cause of cervical and certain other anogenital cancers. Indeed, over 99% of cervical cancers and their precursor cervical intraepithelial neoplasia (CIN) lesions contain HPV DNA. Therefore, vaccination against oncogenic HPV types prevents the development of CIN, and therefore logically, cervical cancer. However, because of the long lead time in the development of cervical cancer, it will take decades for the impact of HPV vaccination on cervical cancer rates to become clear. However, PAP screening programs and ablation of high-grade CIN have successfully reduced the incidence of cervical cancer by approximately 80%. Unfortunately, such screening programs have not been fully implemented in developing countries. As a result, cervical cancer is the second leading killer of women in developing countries. Therefore, the introduction of HPV vaccines globally is of great importance.

The discovery that the major papilloma virus capsid protein (PCP) L1 self-assembles to form virus-like particles (VLPs), which morphologically and antigenically resemble native virions, has revolutionized the HPV vaccine field. The development of vaccines against oncogenic HPVs was further boosted by the demonstration in multiple animal papilloma virus models (rabbits, dogs, and cows) that vaccination with L1 VLPs protects from experimental challenge with the same virus (Chapter 7). There are now two VLP-based vaccines approved for use in humans. Gardasil® is a quadrivalent vaccine that covers two oncogenic HPV types (16 and 18) and two low-risk types (6 and 11), and the bivalent Cervarix® against HPV 16 and 18. The inclusion of HPV6 and HPV11 L1 VLPs offers additional prevention against genital warts.

12.1.1 **L1 VLP vaccines provide type-restricted immunity of unknown duration**

L1 VLP-based vaccines are highly effective; indeed in the landmark phase III prophylactic vaccination trial of HPV16 L1 VLPs, Koutsky *et al.* demonstrated 100% (95% confidence interval, 90–100; $P<0.0001$) protection against acquisition of persistent HPV 16 infection over an 18-month period. Furthermore, the women vaccinated with placebo acquired HPV16+ CIN, whereas those vaccinated with HPV16 VLPs did not. However, both groups acquired similar numbers of CIN, containing genotypes other than HPV 16. This suggested that HPV L1 VLP vaccines provide protection primarily against infection by the homologous papilloma virus type and is consistent with the type restriction of the neutralizing antibody that mediates protection. Furthermore, these findings have been extended in recently published Phase III trials (Chapter 8). Such type-restricted immunity renders comprehensive vaccination against cervical cancer with L1 VLPs extremely difficult. There is also a theoretical concern that the impact of vaccination may wane over time as other genotypes fill the niche created by loss of only two oncogenic genotypes. Importantly, there is evidence of partial cross-protection against types, notably HPV 31 and HPV 45, very closely related to those included in the Gardasil® and Cervarix® vaccines, HPV 16 and HPV 18, respectively. Nevertheless, the protection is only partial and its longevity may be less than that for the homologous HPV type. It is clear that protection against the HPV types targeted by L1 VLP vaccines lasts for at least 5 years. If immunity wanes, then additional boosts or an adjuvant more potent than alum might be necessary.

12.1.2 Highly multivalent HPV L1 VLP vaccines

Perhaps the simplest approach to overcoming the issue of type restriction issue is to increase the valency of the L1 VLP vaccine. For example, a completely effective and type-specific HPV prophylactic vaccine would require 11 distinct formulations to prevent 95.7% of cervical cancer. An octavalent formulation of L1 VLPs of the six most common oncogenic HPV genotypes (HPV 16, HPV 18, HPV 31, HPV 45, HPV 52, and HPV 58) that are responsible for ~90% of cervical cancer cases, as well as the benign types HPV 6 and HPV 11 that cause ~90% of genital warts is being clinically tested. Unfortunately, this increase in valency is also likely to raise the cost of this second-generation HPV vaccine and complexity of manufacture.

12.1.3 Second-generation low-cost HPV L1 VLP vaccines

There are several approaches to reduce the cost of this type of vaccine, which is essential for its worldwide implementation. First, local manufacture, for example, in India, this has been successfully done for the hepatitis B vaccine. Second, alternate production systems such as plants are being explored; this offers the possibility of low-cost manufacture and even avoiding the cost of needles by oral vaccination. L1 VLPs have been successfully produced in tobacco and potato, but further optimization is necessary. Gardasil® is produced in yeast, which is a relatively inexpensive production system and yeast is also potentially edible. Furthermore, nasal immunization with L1 VLPs has shown promise but may require an adjuvant.

12.2 Alternative strategies

12.2.1 HPV L1 capsomere vaccine

125

L1 can be produced to very high levels in *E. coli* as a GST-fusion protein where it accumulates as star-shaped capsomeres that are comprised of five L1 molecules, 72 of which form an intact capsid. Truncation of L1 at its C terminus and mutation of critical cysteine residues prevents the assembly of capsomeres into VLP. The capsomeres alone may not be as immunogenic as VLP, but their immunogenicity was not distinguishable when using an appropriate adjuvant. Importantly, vaccination of dogs with GST-L1 capsomeres protects against viral challenge. Drs R Garcea and R Schlegel are currently developing a GST-HPV16 L1 capsomere vaccine formulated in alum for early phase testing.

12.2.2 **DNA-based vaccines for L1**

Plasmid DNA vaccines offer the potential of low-cost manufacture and temperature stability, and possibly needle-free delivery via 'gene gun' or electroporation. Several groups have shown that vaccination of rabbits with CRPV L1 expression constructs protects against viral challenge. Interestingly, cellular immunity contributes to protection against virus. Vaccination of mice with HPV L1 expression constructs also induces neutralizing antibodies. Potentially, multiple L1 constructs can be co-injected for broad immunity. However, murine studies suggest strong interference when L1 constructs of different types are co-injected, probably because L1 of different types fail to co-assemble into conformationally correct VLPs or differentially compete. Furthermore, while DNA vaccines have been very successful in murine models, delivery of other naked DNA-based vaccines in humans has failed to live up to expectations to date. Furthermore, the specific APCs of the epithelium, Langerhans cells, may differ from other dendritic cells in their ability to recognize L1 VLP, suggesting that simple intradermal vaccination may be problematic.

12.2.3 **Viral vectors for L1**

Live viral systems have been used in animal studies to deliver L1 for vaccination and offer the potential for single dose, low-cost immunization. Vaccination with Vesticular Stomatis virus (VSV) encoded or vaccinia CRPV L1 recombinants protects rabbits from viral challenge. However, immunization with live viral vectors carries more risk than protein vaccines. One approach to address the safety issue is the use of replication defective viral vectors, which are less potent, but more likely to be safe. Vaccination of rhesus macaques with defective adenovirus expressing HPV16 L1 induced significant titers of neutralizing antibodies. But responses to defective viral vectors, like their live counterparts, can be blunted by pre-existing immunity to the viral vector. In addition, neutralizing antibody responses to the vector can limit the potential for boosting responses.

12.2.4 **Bacterial vectors for L1**

Similar to viral vectors, there are a number of potential bacterial vectors for delivery of L1. For example, recombinant BCG expressing CRPV L1 protects rabbits from viral challenge. Another exciting possibility is expression of L1 from attenuated vaccine strains of

Salmonella typhi, which can be readily grown, do not require purification, are generally well tolerated, and are given orally. Oral vaccination offers the possibility of local immunity, although systemic vaccination with VLPs suggests that this is not required for protection. Experiments in mice suggest that L1 delivered by this approach is highly immunogenic, and the antibodies induced are neutralizing. Dr D Nardelli-Haefliger is pursuing clinical testing of this approach.

12.3 **The minor capsid protein L2**

In addition to L1, papilloma viruses have a second minor capsid protein called L2. Figure 12.1 shows the relationship between L1 and L2. L2 is critical for papilloma virus infection, possibly for binding to a secondary viral receptor and facilitating delivery of the viral genome to the nucleus. Importantly, L2 is also a promising alternate antigen for prophylactic vaccination. Indeed, immunization of rabbits or cows with the minor capsid protein L2 or L2 peptides protects from experimental papilloma virus infection at both mucosal and cutaneous sites.

A recent animal study indicates that, as for L1 VLP vaccines, protection against experimental papilloma virus challenge by L2 vaccination is mediated by neutralizing antibodies. However, unlike L1 VLP vaccination, vaccination with HPV L2 induces antibodies that cross-neutralize diverse HPV genotypes (Figure 12.2). We have recently shown that rabbits vaccinated with HPV16 L2 11-200 are protected against experimental viral challenge by two evolutionarily divergent rabbit papilloma viruses CRPV and ROPV. However, these animals grew papillomas when inoculated with CRPV DNA and these papillomas grew at the same rate whether the L2-vaccinated animals were challenged with CRPV wild type DNA or with CRPV DNA defective for L2 expression. This suggests that cell-mediated immunity is not responsible for protection. By contrast, protection was strongly correlated with the induction of even low titres of neutralizing antibodies, suggesting their importance in immunity. We are currently developing a process for the manufacture in *Escherichia coli* of a clinical grade L2 11-200 polypeptide fusion protein derived from multiple HPV types for future clinical testing.

While L1 is highly immunogenic, L2 is immunologically subdominant to L1 in the context of an L1/L2 VLP or virion vaccination as well as in seroepidemiologic studies of natural infection. Therefore, no cross-protection is seen in animals vaccinated with L1/L2 VLPs because they generate only L1-specific neutralizing antibodies (Figure 12.2). This probably reflects the close-packed, regular array of L1, in contrast to L2 which is present in the capsid at a 5- to 30-fold lower level, mostly buried in the capsid vertices and more widely spaced.

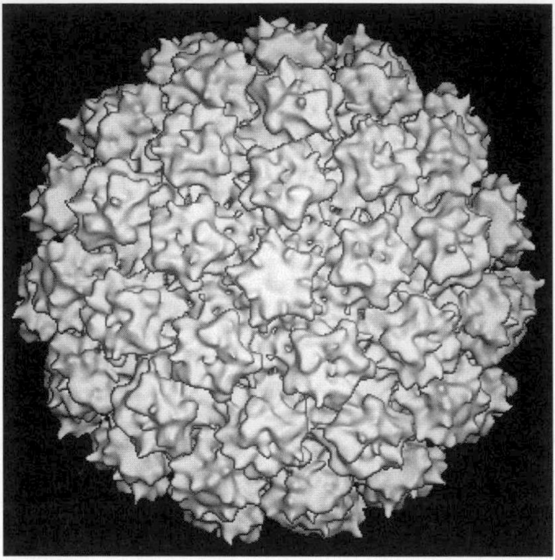

Figure 12.1 A high-resolution image reconstruction of papilloma virus viewed down the 5-fold axis of symmetry.

Trus et al. described the high-resolution structure of bovine papilloma virus (BPV1), using image reconstruction of cryoelectron micrographs. The capsid is non-enveloped and has T=7 icosahedral symmetry. It comprises 72 capsomers, each containing 5 L1 molecules. Sixty capsomers are coordinated with 6 adjacent capsomers (hexavalent) and 12 with five neighbouring capsomers (pentavalent). A pentavalent capsomer can be seen in the centre of this image. The button of density present in the centre of the pentavalent capsomers, and possibly all capsomers, may correspond to the minor capsid protein L2 (although this remains the subject of much debate pending a definitive structural analysis). A small portion of which is exposed on the capsid surface and available for binding by neutralizing antibodies. Image reconstructions of BPV1, HPV1, and CRPV suggest that all papilloma viruses have a very similar structure. The viral genome forms a nucleohistone core with no detectible icosahedral symmetry.

Source: Reproduced from Trus BL et al. . Novel structural features of bovine papilloma virus capsid revealed by a three-dimensional reconstruction to 9Å resolution. *Nature Structure and Molecular Biology*, 4(5): 413–20, (May 2007).

It is likely the virus evolved such that L2 is poorly immunogenic, given its critical conserved role in infection. Otherwise the evolution of the large number of papilloma virus serotypes/genotypes could not have occurred.

Given the weakness of antibody responses to L2 as compared to L1, several groups have attempted display of L2 neutralizing epitopes on the surface of capsids, that is, to make L2 more L1-like. Initial attempts to introduce L2 neutralizing epitopes in the surface immunodominant loops of L1 have been bedeviled by difficulties in main

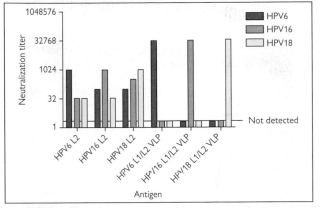

Figure 12.2 Vaccination with L1/L2 VLPs induces type-specific neutralizing antibodies, whereas vaccination with L2 protein alone generates a lower titre, but broadly neutralizing antibody response.

Rabbits were immunized with L1/L2 VLPs or L2 protein alone derived from HPV 6, HPV 16, or HPV 18. Sera were tested for neutralizing titre against HPV 6, HPV 16 or HPV 18 pseudovirions. These HPV types represent prototypic members of three evolutionary clades.

taining efficient assembly, and thus far only low titres of L2-specific neutralization have been produced by immunization with these constructs. Additional efforts to display L2 on better characterized viral capsids, and even in live viral vectors, are ongoing.

12.4 Combining preventive and therapeutic vaccines

Results from ongoing clinical trials demonstrate that vaccination with L1 VLP does not alter the course of pre-existing HPV infection. This likely does not reflect a failure to induce significant L1-specific cell-mediated immunity, but rather the absence of detectable capsid gene expression in the basal epithelial cells that harbour the viral genome. This is also likely to be true of L2 vaccines and preclinical studies in rabbits that bear this out. Therefore, a number of attempts have been made to combine therapeutic efficacy with prophylactic vaccination by fusing early papilloma virus proteins with capsid proteins. Typically the viral early proteins E6 and E7 are targeted because they are required to maintain the transformed state (i.e. they cannot be lost, even in cancer, to evade immunity without triggering cell death). The first example of such a vaccine is TA-CIN, which comprises a fusion of HPV16 L2, E6, and E7 that is generated by bacterial expression. Vaccination with this fusion protein, even without adjuvant, induced

CHAPTER 12 **2nd generation prophylactic vaccines**

both L2-specific neutralizing antibodies and early protein-specific cellular immune responses. However, its ability to protect patients from acquisition of HPV has not been tested. Further, regression of high-grade vaginal/vulval intraepithelial neoplasia (VAIN/VIN) was rarely seen in TA-CIN vaccinated women, even when they were boosted with vaccinia virus expressing E6 and E7 (Chapter 13). Another effort fused E7 to the C-terminus of L1 such that VLP-assembly was maintained. Vaccination of CIN patients with chimeric L1-E7 VLPs induced a robust humoural response to L1, but the clinical response was insufficient to warrant advancement of this vaccine. Nevertheless, there have been significant advances in our understanding of vaccine immunology, adjuvants, and vaccine delivery, and these chimeric HPV vaccines may prove much more potent when delivered with an appropriate adjuvant.

12.5 **Summary**

The demonstrable efficacy of Gardasil® and Cervarix® vaccines has triggered multiple efforts to develop second-generation L1-based vaccines to address some of its shortcomings for global use, notably cost, type restriction, requirement for refrigeration, needle delivery and three immunizations, and inability to induce the clearance of pre-existing infections. Highly multivalent L1 VLP vaccines are currently being evaluated, but cost remains a primary issue preventing global realization of the benefits of HPV vaccination. Several interesting and potentially low-cost candidates will enter the clinical trials shortly, including L1 capsomeres, L2 polypeptide, and *S. typhi* expressing L1.

Further reading

Fraillery D, Baud D, Pang SY, *et al.* (2007). Ty21a expressing human papilloma virus type 16 L1 as a potential live Salmonella vaccine against cervical cancer and typhoid fever. *Clinical Vaccine Immunology*, **14**: 1285–95.

Gambhira R, Jagu S, Karanam B, *et al.* (2007). Protection of rabbits against challenge with rabbit papilloma viruses by immunization with the N-terminus of HPV16 minor capsid antigen L2. *Journal of Virology*, Oct. 10 (Epub) doi.1120/JUI.00936-07.

Koutsky LA, Ault KA, Wheeler CM, *et al.* (2002). A controlled trial of a human papilloma virus type 16 vaccine. *New England Journal of Medicine*, **347**: 1645–51.

Roden R and Wu TC (2006). How will HPV vaccines affect cervical cancer? *National Review of Cancer*, **6**: 753–63.

Villa LL, Costa RL, Petta CA, *et al.* (2005). Prophylactic quadrivalent human papilloma virus (types 6, 11, 16, and 18) L1 virus-like particle vaccine in young women: a randomised double-blind placebo-controlled multicentre phase II efficacy trial. *Lancet Oncology,* **6**: 271–8.

Yuan, Este, PA, Chen Y, *et al.* (2001). Immunization with a pentameric L1 fusion protein protects against papilloma virus infection. *Journal of Virology,* **75**: 7848–53.

Chapter 13

Therapeutic HPV vaccines

Sjoerd H van der Burg

Key points

- Therapeutic vaccines aim to induce or boost HPV T-cell adaptive immunity when it is insufficient or has failed to develop naturally.
- The high-risk HPV type oncogenes E6 and E7 are obligate for driving the malignant process in cervical neoplasia and are the preferred targets.
- Vaccines based on viral protein or peptides together with adjuvants which act to stimulate the desired balance of T-cell response, or naked DNA, viral, or bacterial vectors encoding the viral targets have been tested in preclinical animal models.
- Early phase clinical trials of therapeutic vaccines in cervical cancer patients have shown evidence of immunogenicity and safety, but clinical efficacy has not been established. In part, this is because of the complexity of immunological escape mechanisms which the tumour has utilized during its evolution.
- Trials aimed at treating HPV-persistent infection in recalcitrant VIN 3 are a useful proving ground for testing combined treatment modalities that include vaccination to focus the cellular immunity away from negative influences of T regulatory cells.

13.1 Immune control of cancer

There is now very persuasive evidence that the immune system plays an important part in controlling cancer. There is abundant data documenting immune recognition of tumour antigens (TA) by both T cells and antibodies in animal tumour models and in human cancers. TA can result from genetic changes in the cancer cells such as a chromosomal translocation, mutation, overexpression, or inappropriate expression of molecules related to the process of carcinogenesis, leading to new or abberrantly expressed target epitopes for the immune system, as well as from the expression of viral oncoproteins.

In some cases, lymphocyte infiltration of cancer can be associated with a better prognosis, but if the balance of tumour-infiltrating cells (TIL) favours, for example, T regulatory cells then this can result in a negative outlook for the patient. Expansion ex vivo of TIL and their adoptive transfer into patients has shown some dramatic regressions of tumours and their metastases.

The immune control of malignant disease implies the action of active immune surveillance and the components important to this process have been highlighted by experimental studies in mice, where various aspects of the functioning innate and adaptive immune systems have been deleted genetically and the influence on tumour growth and development assessed. Thus mice lacking specific immune effector cells (T-cells and NK cells), key cytokines (IFN), molecules involved in the processing and presentation of tumour-specific antigens, or molecules of cytotoxic pathways, have a high incidence of tumours or fail to control tumour growth. In particular, dendritic cells (DC), CD4+ T-helper (Th) cells, and CD8+ cytotoxic T-cells (CTL) play an important role in the anti-tumour response (Chapter 6).

Of course when surveillance is successful tumours will not become apparent and when cancers become clinically evident immune surveillance must have been at least partially unsuccessful. Therapeutic cancer vaccines aim to harness the patients' own immune system to revitalize any existing immunity or to induce a new angle of attack, thereby overcoming any tumour-evasion strategies which may be limiting control. Strategies for therapeutic vaccination must identify appropriate TA, maximize their delivery to the professional antigen presenting cells so as to generate the correct balance of T-cell immune effectors, which then need to target the lesions, and overcome any pre-existing negative influences. Importantly, there is very clear evidence from immunosuppressed patients, showing an increased incidence of HPV-induced tumours that directly implicates a role for the immune system in natural control of these types of cancer. Furthermore, studies on the spontaneous immune response against HPV indicate a key role for the HPV-specific T-cell response aimed at the early viral proteins and support the design and development of treatment modalities, which exploit the host's immune system to combat HPV-induced lesions.

13.2 **Vaccine development**

13.2.1 **Target antigens**
The ultimate goal of a therapeutic vaccine would be to successfully treat HPV high-grade lesions and cancers. Treatment of an established (progressive) HPV infection should aim at the enhancement of Th-1

biased/CTL immunity because this is critical for regression of HPV-induced disease (Box 13.1). The viral oncogenes, E6 and E7, are expressed in all of the cells in such premalignant and malignant lesions and thus have been selected as prime targets for vaccine development. Evidence from spontaneous immune responses in experimental animal models of natural infection and in human beings suggest that the early antigens E2 and E6 form the target antigens for clearance of both persistent infection and low-grade lesions.

13.2.2 Vaccine design

The viral target antigen can be delivered as a protein, as DNA, encoded in a bacterial or viral vector or in DC loaded with antigen. In all these examples the vaccine aims to maximize the stimulation of the appropriate T-cell responses and each system has potential advantages and disadvantages. Different approaches mimic or interface with the natural antigen processing and presentation pathways of the immune system, accompanied by appropriate danger signals. Proteins, peptides, and DNA generally lack danger signals and this is compensated for by co-delivery of adjuvants. Viral-vectors usually inherently contain adjuvant properties. An adjuvant enhances the immunity to the vaccine target antigen and an understanding of such effects offers new approaches to successful vaccine development. All vaccines must then be tested in preclinical animal models before they can be

---

Box 13.1 An ideal candidate therapeutic vaccine

- Displays excellent safety profile, is easy to prepare, and can be used 'off the shelf'.
- Can be used in all patients regardless of tissue type (HLA).
- Is highly immunogenic but does not compete with the antigen of interest for the attention of the immune system.
- Does not evoke neutralizing antibodies, which may limit the number of booster injections.
- Targets the early proteins expressed in the lesions, including E2, E6, and E7 which makes it possible to use it at several stages of disease (post-infection, persistent infection, LGSIL, HGSIL, and cancer).
- Induces both a strong CD4+ T-helper cell type 1 and a CD8+ cytotoxic T-cell-mediated immune effector response to ensure the long-term presence of activated immune effector cells.
- Ensures that activated HPV-specific T-cells migrate to their target-cell tissue.
- Results in long-term HPV-specific memory (especially when given as treatment at early stages of disease) to prevent reappearance of HPV-induced lesions.
- Displays cross-protective immunity to other high-risk types of HPV.
- Generates immunity able to overcome local immunosuppression, limiting issues such as T regulatory cells or impaired antigen presentation by the tumour.

tested in humans. A number of candidate immunotherapeutic vaccines aiming at the induction of HPV antigen-specific immunity have been developed during the past years (Table 13.1).

Protein vaccines: Viral proteins can be produced by cloning the genes into various bacterial expression systems and then purifying the molecules to homogeneity. It is also possible to genetically engineer more than one protein into a fusion product. This is possible because the protein needs to be processed by antigen presenting cells and appropriately activate the specific T-cells. Alternatively, peptide fragments which can bind to particular HLA molecules to form the complex recognized by specific T-cell receptors have been used. The first generation of peptide vaccines were based on selected CTL and/or Th cell epitopes able to bind to only one HLA molecule. This severely restricted their use in large groups of patients. A second generation of peptide vaccines constitutes longer peptides, which are predominantly presented by professional APC and as a consequence are highly immunogenic and capable of fully activating T-cell responses. When injected as pools of overlapping peptides, covering a complete antigen sequence, the problem of HLA restriction is

Table 13.1 Therapeutic HPV16 vaccines tested

Vaccine type	Patient type	Vaccine-induced E6–E7 immunity
CTL Peptide (E7)	CC (end stage)	No
CTL Peptide (E7)	CIN2/3 and VIN3	Yes, CD8 (~55%)
Long peptide pools (E6 & E7)	CC (end stage) CC (after surgery)	Yes (>80%) Yes, CD4 & CD8 (100%)
Fusion protein (L2E6E7)	Normal	Yes (~75%)
Fusion protein (E6E7 + ISCOMATRIX	CIN	Yes, CD4 (~80%) + CD8 (~35%)
hspE7	CIN3	Yes CD4 (15%)
PD-E7	CIN1/3	Yes, CD4 & CD8 (~30%)
cVLP (L1E7)	CIN2/3	Yes (~25%)
Vaccinia (E6E7)	CC (early stage) VIN3	Yes, CD8 (15%) Yes (~50%)
Encapsulated DNA (E6E7 fragments)	CIN2/3	Yes (~40%)
DC (E7)	CC (end stage)	Yes (~30%)
DC (E7) + IL-2	CC (end stage)	Yes, CD4 (50%) & CD8 (75%)

CC: patients with cervical cancer, Normal: healthy individual with no sign of HPV infection or disease.

solved. Similar to the synthetic long peptides vaccines, protein vaccines are not restricted by HLA type but lack the properties to endow DC with the activating signals needed to induce a strong CTL response. Both types of vaccines depend on the development of CD4+ T-cell responses to provide such signals to DC. The use of adjuvants, mixed or fused to the peptides or proteins, strongly enhances their immunogenicity and efficacy. In addition, immunogenicity is optimized via the enhancement of antigen delivery by encapsulation of proteins and peptides, using (a) virosomes of influenza virus, (b) ISCOM's, cage-like immunostimulating structures, (c) liposomes, or (d) fused to the late proteins of HPV 16 as chimeric virus-like particles (cVLPs). The idea behind the latter is that cVLP induces HPV16 L1-specific antibodies and, therefore, work as both a prophylactic and therapeutic vaccine.

DNA vaccines: While peptide and protein vaccines are safe and relatively easy to produce, it is also possible to inject the DNA encoding the viral sequences directly. Such naked DNA vaccines are very cheap to produce although modification to the viral oncogenes to limit their function need to be made, but there are no restrictions with respect to HLA types of the vaccinees. DNA vaccines display a low immunogenicity because only those cells expressing this DNA can produce the target antigen and the DNA itself cannot amplify or spread in vivo unlike viruses or bacteria. Current DNA vaccination strategies rely on multiple intramuscular or intradermal injections. DNA vaccines primarily stimulate CD8+ T-cell responses but can be constructed to induce CD4 T-cell responses. To improve delivery and antigenicity, encapsulation of DNA in biodegradable particles or delivery via tattooing is an option.

Viral and bacterial vector vaccines: Viral and bacterial vectors expressing the modified viral oncogenes are easy to prepare, but there are always safety concerns. The vectors themselves are highly immunogenic which is advantageous since a strong Th1/CTL response towards the encoded viral tumour-antigen is required, but can also be a significant drawback because the immune system may rather focus its T- and B-cell responses to antigens of the vector itself, with the risk of inducing non-relevant T-cells or vector-specific antibodies that could limit the value of booster injections. One strategy to minimize this is to use different vaccine vehicles encoding the TA in the first (prime) and second (boost) immunizations. Other advantages are the production of large quantities of TA available for processing and presentation by the immune system, accompanied by highly relevant danger signals. Most widely used are recombinant vaccinia viruses expressing E6 and E7. Other vectors include recombinant Semliki Forest virus, Venezuelan equine encephalitis, virus replicon particle vaccines, and the bacterial vectors Listeria Monocytogenes, Salmonella, Shigella, and Escherichia coli.

Dendritic cell vaccines: DCs are the professional antigen-presenting cells which have a strong capacity to stimulate T-cells and can be prepared from individual patients' peripheral blood monocytes. DC-based therapy requires the preparation of a new product for each patient. So far DC-vaccine induced immunity is not optimal and needs improvement with respect to antigen loading, maturation, and administration. Several vehicles, including viral vectors, tumour lysates, transfection with mRNA, peptides, and proteins have been used to load antigens. Migration of intradermally administered mature DCs to the draining lymph nodes, which in the mouse correlates with T-cell proliferation, is low, implying that migration needs to be optimized. Currently employed strategies include pretreatment of the vaccine injection site with inflammatory compounds.

Animal models testing: Murine tumours expressing HPV genes have provided accessible models for the preclinical testing and optimization of HPV-specific therapeutic vaccines. However, the growth of such transplantable murine tumours differs significantly from the natural development of papilloma virus-induced tumours and, therefore, while most therapeutic strategies have been validated using such studies the insight for human disease is somewhat limited. The dog and rabbit papilloma virus models more closely resemble high-risk HPV infections with the development of viral persistence and associated malignancies and these have been utilized. Similar to human models, progression is in part genetically determined and linked to their HLA tissue type background. Most vaccine approaches were able to successfully alter the course of disease in a setting where the vaccine was injected at subclinical stages of disease. In a few cases the successful eradication of established warts were reported, implying that therapeutic vaccination can be used to effectively treat individuals with persistent HPV infections as well as HPV-induced LSIL.

The development of therapeutic vaccines in cancer is still at an early stage and as our understanding of the immunological details improves it will be possible to get closer to the requirements of an 'ideal therapeutic vaccine' (Box 13.1).

13.3 **HPV16 vaccines in human trials**

Following preclinical testing, several therapeutic vaccines have been tested in early phase clinical trials. These are concerned with safety and proof of concept (e.g. do the vaccines induce T-cell responses in the patients) and are generally not powered to account clinical efficacy.

13.3.1 Peptide and protein vaccines

The first trial with a peptide-based vaccine involved the injection of two HPV16 E7 encoded HLA-A*0201-restricted CTL peptide-epitopes, but no immunological response to the CTL peptides was observed. In a second trial such CTL peptide-epitopes were injected into patients with high-grade lesions of the cervix, with 10/18 patients showing a vaccine-induced T-cell response, but there was no correlation with clinical responses (Table 13.1). This was no surprise if only because this type of vaccine failed to induce the regression of tumours in the mouse model. Recently, the capacity of a HPV16 E6E7 synthetic long peptides (SLP) vaccine was tested in patients with cervical cancer. This vaccine displayed an excellent performance in head-to-head comparison studies with the minimal CTL peptide-epitope. SLP vaccines showed far greater immunogenicity, displayed more favourable pharmacokinetics, and sustained the CTL response for a long time. Prime-boost vaccinations resulted in the regression of established tumours in mice and resulted in regression of established warts in the rabbit papilloma virus model. More than 80% of end-stage cervical cancer patients injected with the HPV16 E6E7 SLP vaccine displayed a broad HPV16-specific immune response, consisting of both CD4+ Th1/Th2 cells and CD8+ T-cells. Co-injection of the E6 and E7 peptides resulted in an E6-focused response, while the injection of E6 and E7 peptides at distinct sites resulted in strong reactivity to both E6 and E7.

The immunogenicity and efficacy of several protein vaccines have been tested in the clinic, but none of them in patients with cancer (Table 13.1). An HPV16 L2E6E7 fusion protein vaccine (TA-CIN) induced a protective CTL response in mice and induced both L2 antibody responses and (E6-focused) T-cell responses in 75% of vaccinated healthy volunteers. Another protein vaccine, in which HPV16 E7 was fused to heat-shock protein, serving as in-built adjuvant, induced tumour regression in mice but was not able to induce/enhance HPV-specific immunity in patients, despite the fact that pre-existing HPV16-specific CD4+ T-cell responses were detected in half of the patients. The observed clinical regressions were not correlated with immunity or clearance of HPV. Similarly, when HPV16 E7 was fused to H. Influenza protein D only few HPV16 CIN3 patients responded specifically to E7. The injection of an HPV16L1E7 cVLP vaccine induced an L1-specific antibody response in all vaccinated HPV16+ CIN2/3 patients whereas the response rate to E7 was poor. No significant clinical response is observed which correlates well with the outcome of the large field studies in which no therapeutic effect of the prophylactic vaccine (L1-VLP) on established infections was observed. Interestingly, the HPV16 E6E7 fusion protein with ISCOMATRIX adjuvant was highly immunogenic in patients with

CIN1 to CIN3. In 80% of the patients CD4+ T-cell reactivity was detected against E6, and in 50% against E7. Notably, the E6 response was stronger and earlier. CD8+ T-cell responses were detected in 35% of the patients.

13.3.2 DNA vaccines

A DNA vaccine, encoding fragments of HPV16/18 E6 and E7, which potentially may induce cross-reactive T-cells, was encapsulated in biodegradable particles (ZYC101) and induced a HPV16-specific T-cell response in 40% of women with CIN2/3. Clinical responses were not associated with immunity or lack thereof, nor with HPV type (Table 13.1).

13.3.3 Viral vector vaccines

Several trials have been performed in patients with cervical cancer, using vaccinia viruses (used to eradicate smallpox) engineered to express HPV16/18 E6 and E7 (TA-HPV). The vaccine was safe and able to induce HPV-specific T-cell reactivity in some patients, but also induced vaccinia-specific antibodies. In attempts to investigate efficacy, patients with high-grade lesions of the vulva (VIN) were treated in two trials. Clinical responses, defined as shrinkage of the size of the lesion by more than 50%, as well as HPV16-specific T-cell immunity (focused to E6) were observed in about half of the patients. When the results of these trials were combined, the number of clinical responders was significantly higher in the patient group displaying vaccine-induced HPV16-specific type 1 T-cell immunity compared with those who failed to mount such a response; unfortunately no clear-cut associations between immunity and clinical efficacy could be determined. Based on the experiments in a mouse tumour model showing that the immune response may be improved by a vaccination scheme in which first a protein-based vaccine (TA-CIN) was injected, followed by a vaccinia-based vaccine (TA-HPV), such a heterologous prime-boost protocol has also been tested in patients with high-grade VIN. Although successful in mice, again about half of the patients displayed an immune response, which again was focused on E6, and this response was predominantly induced/boosted by TA-HPV and not by TA-CIN (Table 13.1).

Recombinant modified vaccinia virus Ankara (MVA) is considered to be safer than other vaccinia virus constructs and has been used to express E2 of bovine papilloma virus. Direct injection of this vaccine into the uterus of patients with HPV16/18+ CIN2/3, once a week for 6 weeks, resulted in a significant number of eliminated lesions, probably due to strong T-cell reactivity against the vaccinia virus injected in the lesions.

13.3.4 DC vaccines

DC-based vaccines protected mice against the outgrowth of a transplantable tumour and have also been tested in patients with advanced cervical cancer. In a trial where DCs pulsed with E7 protein was injected, about 30% of the patients showed evidence of an E7-specific immune response. This percentage increased in another trial in which E7-pulsed DCs were injected in combination with IL-2 (Table 13.1). No clinical responses were observed.

13.4 Trial design

As yet, there is no ideal vaccine (strategy) and, therefore, most of the trials were of an exploratory type with safety and immunogenicity as primary endpoints. With respect to the immunogenicity of HPV-specific vaccines two points need to be considered: (1) the presence of wrongly polarized HPV16-specific T-cells (Th2 cells, regulatory T-cells) urges trials of HPV16-specific vaccines to be performed in HPV16-positive patients. Vaccination of patients with other HPV-types, and as such with a 'naïve' T-cell repertoire to HPV16, may overestimate the immunological outcome, and (2) both E6 and E7 are the key target antigens for immunotherapy and are in general incorporated into a single vaccine. Earlier studies reveal a dominance of E6-specific reactivity over the T-cell response against E7. Thus, in new trials the induction of E7-specific immunity requires attention. Ultimately, the most promising candidate vaccine approaches will need to be tested in placebo-controlled trials, testing them against best practice treatment and powered to detect some real clinical value.

Clinical efficacy is generally assessed using conventional tumour response endpoints, which measure tumour/lesion reduction/size (RECIST criteria). Such definitions of response may be useful in assessing treatment of persistent infections (no HPV DNA detectable), pre-malignant disease (regression of lesion), or when used as adjuvant therapy after surgery (no recurrences). It is debatable whether such criteria are always the most relevant to define useful clinical responses in patients with cancer. In other types of cancers, immunotherapy and other treatments have sometimes resulted in significant increases in progression-free survival or overall survival in absence of clear tumour regression. Such an endpoint may also be applicable in therapeutic vaccination trials of cervical cancer.

13.5 Future prospects

While it is likely that the response rate of patients with HPV-induced high-grade lesions or cancer to therapeutic vaccines will never reach

100%, substantial benefits may be gained by combining vaccines with other therapeutic regimens. Immune escape, HPV-specific regulatory T-cells, and a hostile local microenvironment represent a number of immunotherapeutic hurdles (Table 13.2) for which potential solutions need to be sought. Many of the 'solutions' described in the following section are currently being evaluated in humans (see Figure 13.1). The use of immune potentiating compounds (e.g. Toll-like receptor ligands, cytokine-antibody complexes, agonistic antibodies to co-stimulatory molecules) and/or antagonistic antibodies to co-inhibitory receptors (CTLA-4, PD1) will ascertain a stronger stimulation of effective Th1/CTL-type responses and may even tip the balance between regulatory T-cells and effector T-cells towards the latter. Indeed, removal of pre-existing regulatory T-cells significantly

Table 13.2 Hurdles in successful immunotherapy

Hurdle	Effect on immunity
• Lack of local inflammation attention	• Failure to attract immune systems • No active migration of immune cells to lesion
• Lack of cell death	• No sufficient cross-presentation of viral proteins to activate strong HPV-specific T-cells responses
• Modulated presentation of viral peptides target	• Difficulties for T-cells to recognize and destroy cells
• Down regulation of HLA at cell surface	• Activation of T-cells not able to recognize HPV positive cells anymore • Escape of HPV-positive cells from immunity
• Expression of anti-apoptotic proteins cells	• Recognized target cells are rescued from killer cells
• Immunosuppressive local environment	• Conversion of APC towards a type that is non-supportive for Th1/CTL immunity • Dysregulation and/or suppression of immune effector function in lesion
• Presence of regulatory T-cells	• Failure to activate/expand HPV-specific T-cell response in lesion draining lymph nodes • Down regulation of immune effector function in lesion • Pre-existent HPV-specific regulatory T-cells can be expanded by vaccines resulting in further down regulation of immunity

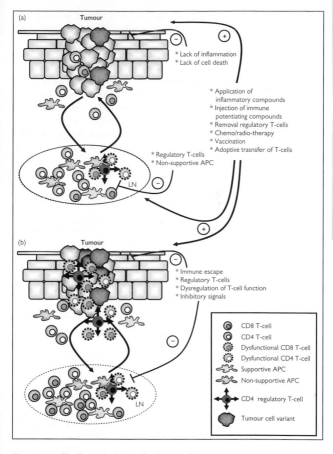

Figure 13.1 Hurdles and solutions for the use of therapeutic vaccination in the immunotherapy of HPV-induced lesions and cancers.

The extent of immune infiltration differs between each and every tumour and ranges from almost none (a) to extensive (b). The inherent lack of inflammation of most tumours, a non-supportive milieu and the presence of regulatory T-cells in tumour draining lymph nodes may provide an explanation for a failure of the immune system to infiltrate the lesion, whereas immune escape, through the expression of anti-apoptotic molecules or modulation of HLA class I peptide presentation, and inhibitory signals from tumour cells or tumour infiltrating regulatory T-cells, resulting in the conversion of effector T-cells into dysfunctional cells may explain why strongly infiltrated tumours are not controlled (–). These hurdles may be overcome through the combination of several treatments (+).

improves vaccine-induced T-cell responses in mice and humans, and can be achieved by treatment with low doses of cyclophosphamide. Homing of T-cells to cervical lesions and tumours is essential but often fails due to immunosuppressive mechanisms. Combinations of vaccines with treatment modalities able to induce pro-inflammatory signals, either induced by chemotherapy, radiation, or by topical application of creams that contain TLR ligands, are likely to successfully recruit effector T-cells. Tumour escape, through defects in the HLA class I-restricted antigen presentation pathway, may be avoided by the activation of CTL which recognize an alternative repertoire of peptides presented by the HLA molecules of cells with impaired function of molecules associated with antigen processing. Last but not least, an increasing number of reports indicating that radiotherapy and chemotherapy appear more effective in patients with solid tumours who previously received a form of immunotherapy. In mice, HPV16+ tumours regressed more rapidly by adoptively transferred CTL after chemo-/radiotherapy. In addition, the combination of DNA vaccination with chemotherapy led to higher cure rates.

Further reading

Hildesheim A (2007). Effect of human papilloma virus 16/18 L1 viruslike particle vaccine among young women with preexisting infection: a randomized trial. *Journal of American Medical Association*, **298**: 743–53.

Mocellin S (2004). Part I: Vaccines for solid tumours. *Lancet Oncology*, **5**: 681–9.

Schlom J (2007). Cancer vaccines: moving beyond current paradigms. *Clinical Cancer Research,* **1**(13): 3776–82.

van der Burg SH (2006). Improved peptide vaccine strategies, creating synthetic artificial infections to maximize immune efficacy. *Advanced Drug Delivery Reviews*, **58**: 916–30.

van der Burg SH (2007). Cervical cancer is associated with the presence of CD4+ regulatory T-cells specific for the high risk human papilloma virus E6 oncoprotein. *Proceedings of the National Academy of Sciences, USA*, **104**: 12087–92.

van Hall T (2006). Selective cytotoxic T-lymphocyte targeting of tumor immune escape variants. *National Medicine*, **12**: 417–24.

Wang E (2005). Understanding the response to immunotherapy in humans. *Springer Semin Immunopathology*, **27**: 105–17.

Zou W (2006). Regulatory T cells, tumour immunity and immunotherapy. *National Review of Immunology*, **6**: 295–307.

Chapter 14

Conclusion

Peter L Stern and Henry C Kitchener

The development of prophylactic human papilloma virus (HPV) vaccines and proof of efficacy as described in this book represents a landmark in the field of preventative medicine. The challenge now is to implement use of these vaccines and in so doing to see a significant impact on incidence and death rates from cervical cancer. This needs to be most effectively achieved in resource-poor countries, where cancer rates are higher but obstacles to vaccine implementation will be greatest. Unfortunately, in a world of competing healthcare priorities, having the means and know how does not always translate into success. This is well illustrated in 'Safe Motherhood', where appalling rates of maternal mortality persist in sub-Saharan Africa and parts of Asia. Let us hope that political will can be matched with affordability and resources being made available so that a preventable cancer, which currently kills 250000 women annually, can be controlled. Factors that can assist in achieving this goal include: 1) public health recommendations in developing countries that prioritize generalized vaccination of adolescents. 2) The pre-qualification by WHO for HPV vaccines that can be purchased by UN agencies. WHO provides a service to UNICEF and other UN agencies that purchase vaccines, and determines the acceptability in principle of vaccines from different sources for supply to these agencies. There is an established procedure used by WHO for the initial evaluation of candidate vaccines. Reassessment at regular intervals ensures the continuing quality of vaccines currently being supplied. 3) Endorsement of HPV vaccination by the GAVI Alliance. This is a global health partnership representing stakeholders in immunisation from both private and public sectors: developing world and donor governments, private sector philanthropists such as the Bill & Melinda Gates Foundation, the financial community, developed and developing country vaccine manufacturers, research and technical institutes, civil society organisations and multilateral organisations like the World Health Organization (WHO), the United Nations Children's Fund (UNICEF) and the World Bank. The mission is to accelerate access to existing underused vaccines, strengthen health and immunisation systems in countries and introduce innovative new immunisation technology, including vaccines.

Even where HPV vaccine will be available, implementation needs to address some serious issues. Foremost is education, so that women and their daughters understand the potential benefit of primary prevention. Despite the success of screening, around 20% of women do not access screening for a variety of reasons, and this is particularly true in younger women. Among the 'hard to reach' groups are socio-economically deprived women, those from ethnic minorities, and of course, there are anxious individuals who just cannot cope with the idea of cervical screening. We need to ensure that this is not duplicated with vaccination. The public provision of these vaccines should ensure that all girls in the United Kingdom are vaccinated but the attitude of their parents, who will need to consent, will be critical. Separating the primary purpose of a cancer-preventing vaccine from HPV as a sexually transmitted infection will be key in optimizing its acceptability for certain groups.

Although vaccination will reduce cervical cancer risk by at least 70% (the actual proportion could be higher due to cross protection provided there is high uptake of vaccination in the population) screening will remain important and this message needs to be well understood by younger women who currently have the lowest rates of cervical screening coverage. The screening programme itself faces challenges over the next 10 years since the case for replacing cytology as the primary test becomes more compelling. Any major changes to screening will need to be very carefully managed as women trust the 'smear test' or 'PAP test' and any move to HPV testing may have unintended consequences.

Two licensed vaccines have shown some cross-protection against other HPV 16- and 18-related types associated with cervical neoplasia, potentially contributing to increased efficacy in preventing cervical neoplasia. Although efficacy against 'all type' CIN2+ can be determined from large vaccine trials, it may not be possible to document the precise degree of cross-protection in preventing high grade CIN related to less common HPV types, simply because of limited statistical power. It may therefore be necessary to accept prevention of persistent infection by these less frequent types as a relevant endpoint to assess broader type specific cross protection. In countries such as UK and Australia with national vaccination programmes, linking vaccination and screening databases at the level of individual women will be essential in determining the impact of vaccination in preventing cervical abnormalities, as well as providing a rational basis for adjustments to screening algorithms.

There is considerable interest in understanding the relevance of antibody levels to prevention of infection and disease. Apart from the different VLPs, the two vaccines are formulated with different adjuvants, which are included to boost the immune response in terms of antibody levels and longevity of responses. A recent comparative study (Einstein et al, 2009) has provided some insight into the comparative immune responses to the bivalent and quadrivalent vaccines using a virus neutralising assay, which approximates to true neutralisation as the likely method of vaccine protection. The bivalent vaccine induced higher levels of both HPV16 and 18 neutralising antibodies after the third dose in women aged 18–45 years. The higher levels of HPV 18 antibodies induced by the bivalent vaccine compared to the quadrivalent one may explain the observed cross protection against type 45 related CIN2+, already referred to in Chapter 8. Antibody levels are likely to be important for sustained vaccine protection, but the precise requirements (immune correlate of protection) will only become clearer with time. New vaccine candidates which contain multiple high risk HPV types designed to prevent 90% of cancer would need to be tested in trials to demonstrate their superior efficacy. Further refinements in the use of adjuvants could be critical in achieving antibody levels affording useful (cross) protection and longevity. These could allow for using reduced amounts of immunogen and/or the number of immunisations, and have important implications for future boost requirements and timing. As already stated, a critical issue which can only be clarified over time, is the duration of vaccine protection. It will take 15–20 years before a vaccinated girl reaches an age when cervical cancer becomes a significant risk and by that time we need to know whether booster vaccination will be required.

While the current generation of vaccines may prevent a significant proportion CIN3, a considerable amount of high-grade CIN will inevitably occur for many years to come. A therapeutic vaccine to treat a persistent HPV infection, or even CIN2+, would be an important advance in reducing morbidity, but much progress is required to achieve significant clinical efficacy at a level that can challenge current therapy.

The global community of multidisciplinary research scientists and clinicians will continue to work with each other and with the pharmaceutical industry to overcome these hurdles, and we must hope that vaccination can save as many, if not more, lives over the next 30 years as screening has achieved over the last 30 years.

Further reading

Einstein MH, Baron M, Levin MJ, Chatterjee A, Edwards RP, Zepp F, Carletti I, Dessy FJ, Trofa AF, Schuind A, Dubin G. Comparison of the immunogenicity and safety of Cervarix(®) and Gardasil(®) human papillomavirus (HPV) cervical cancer vaccines in healthy women aged 18–45 years. Hum Vaccin. 2009;5(10), 1–15.

http://www.gavialliance.org/resources/16_HPV_Landscape_Jun08.pdf

http://www.who.int/immunization_standards/vaccine_quality/pq_system/en/index.html

Index

153